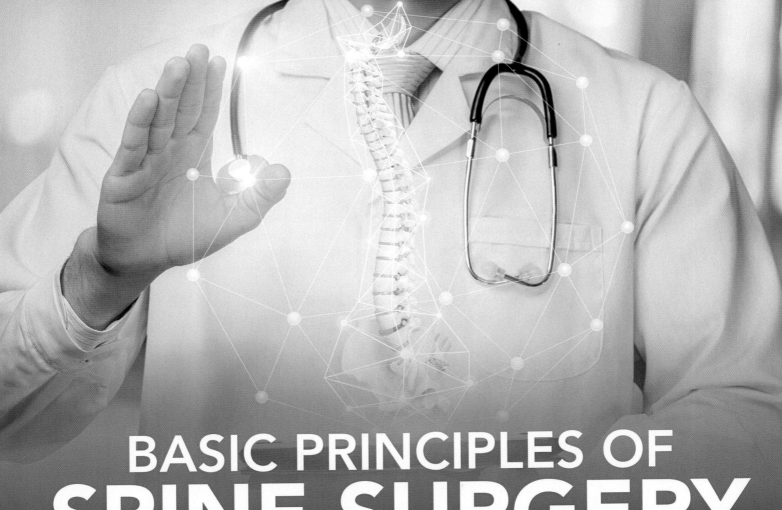

THAMER AHMED HAMDAN
SAAD JUMAAH ABDULSALAM

BASIC PRINCIPLES OF
SPINE SURGERY
ETHICS

AuthorHouse™ UK
1663 Liberty Drive
Bloomington, IN 47403 USA
www.authorhouse.co.uk
UK TFN: 0800 0148641 (Toll Free inside the UK)
UK Local: 02036 956322 (+44 20 3695 6322 from outside the UK)

Because of the dynamic nature of the Internet, any web addresses or links contained in this book may have changed since publication and may no longer be valid. The views expressed in this work are solely those of the author and do not necessarily reflect the views of the publisher, and the publisher hereby disclaims any responsibility for them.

Any people depicted in stock imagery provided by Getty Images are models, and such images are being used for illustrative purposes only.
Certain stock imagery © Getty Images.

This book is printed on acid-free paper.

ISBN: 978-1-7283-5433-0 (sc)
ISBN: 978-1-7283-5432-3 (e)

Print information available on the last page.

Published by AuthorHouse   09/25/2020

authorHOUSE®

Dedication

This book is dedicated to spine surgeons all over the globe, interested in ethics, and consider ethics as important as the surgical technique. It's also dedicated to Lord and Lady Swinfen, for their outstanding service for human beings all over the globe.

Preface

Ethics is considered of prime importance in all aspect of medicine, but it's really much more in spine practice, due to the rapid development of spinal fixator and instrumentations to buy the brains of the spine surgeons to their benefit.

Research and innovation in spine surgery is rapidly developing, which is very vital to improve spine practice, and here again, ethics is very much required.

We carry very special respect to the spine surgeons who are strong believer in implanting the ethical bases in spine practice.

The motivation behind writing this book is the decline in the application of the ethical conduct all over the globe.

Up to our knowledge, there is no similar book in in English language, emphasizing the importance of ethics in spine surgery.

This book is intended for spine surgeons whether they are orthopedic or neurosurgeons, for the residents, and post graduate students.

It contains several chapters, covering almost all aspect of ethical conduct, starting from history, and ending in ethics committee, written in a simple, clear, and understandable language, hopefully, this book will provide key opportunities to improve not only patient care, but also spine surgery as a field of specialty.

Moreover, provide guidance to avoid the pressure of the companies to drive the outcome of surgery and research to their benefit.

Finally, we would like to express our gratitude to those who wrote in the field of ethics, and their writings were very helpful to write this book.

Wrong is wrong, even if everyone is doing it. Right is right even if no one is doing it.

Thamer A. Hamdan
Saad J. Abdulsalam

Contents

Introduction

Ethically, every surgeon should be??

Ethics is defined as moral principles covers a person's behavior or the conducting of an activity, or the branch of knowledge that deals with moral principles. It's a branch of philosophy that that involve systematizing, defending, and recommending concepts of right and wrong conduct. The ethics was found in Hammurabi rules (Babylon) 2000 BC, then followed by Hippocratic Oath, prayer of Moses Maimonides, Geneva declaration, Helsinki codes, AMA code of medical ethics, and all Holly books insist on the ethical points.

The ethics in general is governed by the four principles, which is respect for; autonomy, beneficence, non-maleficence, and justice. To these points, we add the respect for dignity of the patient.

Ethics start from the humanitarian handling of the patient in the first visit, with a big smile, and smooth welcoming words, a lot of respect, careful listening and understanding, followed by very gentle physical examination. If investigations or imaging required, it should be addressed to the specified places, far away from the exchange of personal benefits, and it should be absolutely indicated. In mind, the patients' financial status and away from the laboratory and hospital benefits.

Think always how to alleviate the patients' suffering, rather than how much to gain from him, because the patients' benefit should come at the top of everything. After achieving the definitive diagnosis, everything must be clarified to the patient in a gentle way, particularly, if a serious condition discovered. The informed consent, which is part of the ethical conduct, must contain every details, including the complications and the prognosis.

A gentle communication skills is required to deliver the bad news, the treatment is to be tailored solely for the patients' specific condition, faraway from hospital or companies benefits.

Prescribing narcotic drugs better to be as least as possible, to reduce the risk of addiction.

Justice is required in treating all patients equally, even if they are war prisoners. No difference related to race, color, religion, gender, discrimination, and believe.

Negligence is a surgical crime.

Second opinion is considered mandatory if required, and it's much better than wrong medical service.

Running between hospitals, make the surgeon mentally busy, and it's reflected badly on the service offered, because of this situation, some surgeons leave the follow up to the junior staff, which is reflected badly on the patients' moral. Moreover, some pathology may be missed by the junior staff. Sadly some surgeons insist on using certain implants or medicines, irrespective to the price, with the intension of benefit exchange, which is ethically rejected.

What is worse than this, is performing surgery for no indication, except making the surgeons' pocket heavier, or for the benefit of the private hospital.

Another point of weakness, is to make operative decision depending on the results of investigations or imaging, forgetting the false positive results. On the other hand, no surgery done because the patient cannot offer the money required. This policy should be resisted, and the surgeons' duty is to find avenue to help the poor patients.

Globally, there is over utilization of surgery for many reasons, probably, on the top of this is the financial gain of the surgeons. Failure of conservative treatment is not always a good indication of surgery. The outcome of recent advances is better to be considered cautiously, until it stands the test of time, so we have to wait for the foam to settle down.

The juniors have the right to learn, and improve their technical skills, but this should be done under strict supervision.

There is ethical rules governing the funding of clinical trials from the market companies, so that bias can be avoided.

Also there is ethical rules protecting the patients, and even experimental animal rights, for performing research.

It is a good idea to ask the patient to appoint a proxy, to give permission for procedures not agreed upon prior to surgery, but discovered to be necessary at the time of surgery.

Unfortunately, some surgeons try to push the patient away when bad outcomes or complications developed, we feel the contrary, that the surgeon should help his patient, and find a solution in this desperate situation.

Finally, we look for a good surgeon, who is frank, honest, far away from the financial gain, respect the patient, and never give a false sense of hope, with sound skills, judgment, and full of ethics.

I. History of Medical Ethics

Concern for medical ethics has been expressed since the beginning of human history in the form of laws, decrees, assumptions and "oaths" prepared for or by physicists. Among the oldest are the Hammurabi Code in Babylon (about 1750 BCE), Egyptian papyrus, Indian and Chinese writings and early Greek writers, most notably Hippocrates (lived between 460 and 377 BCE)[1].

The classical example of this poetic expression is the history and evolution of the philosophy of medical ethics. Virtually, each human culture has some supernatural powers to justify the root of morality. Since its very birth Indian ethics had been metaphysical. Ethics was an important part of metaphysical and theological thought about the essence of truth in the Vedas (1500 B.C.). The Vedas explains how people should live and is the world's oldest literature of philosophy. It was the first account in human history of the theological ethics. The old Testament of (c.200 B.C.) the Hebrew Bible (Greek- ta biblia – "the books) gives account of God giving the Ten Commandments – the oral and written Law engraved on tablets of Stone to Moses around 13th

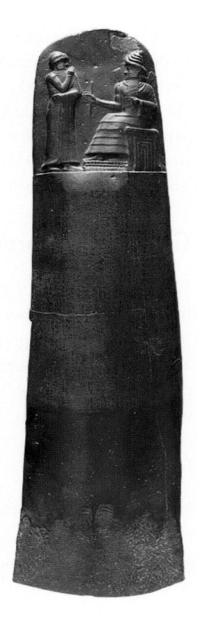

century B.C. on Mount Sinai (Arabic – Gebel Musa) the Mountain near the tip of the Sinai Peninsula in West Asia [1-3].

Early medical ethical codes were written by individuals or by small groups of people, usually physicians. The Oath of Hippocrates is considered historically to be the first such code written in an organized and logical way which describes the proper relationships between physician and patient. During the Middle Ages, other medical codes were written. In recent times, Thomas Precival's writings, disseminated in 1803, represent one of the first ethical codes in the United States and the Western world [1-3].

Code of Hammurabi: Code of Ethics

Hammurabi (1728 – 1686 B.C.) was the Sixth King of the first dynasty of Babylon in Mesopotamia (present Iraq). He was a great ruler, and powerful. Throughout his time he made the Supreme of Babylon. During his rule, he instituted mathematical and astrological treatises and dictionaries. The Sun God Shamash allegedly presented Hammurabi with the code of laws. The Legal Code contains 282 laws which regulate society, family life, and economic activity. The code is etched on a 2 meter high stele found in 1901 in Susa, Iran, and currently stored in the famous Louvre Museum in Paris, France.

Medical Ethics requires guidelines for doctors to act. The medical fees related to the patient's social level. Punished by punitive legislation were misconduct and neglect. "If a physician has performed a major operation upon a lord with a bronze lancet and has saved his life, he shall receive ten shekels of silver, but if he caused the death of such a notable, his hand would be chopped off. A doctor causing the death of a slave would have to replace him." [5].

Babylon was the wealthy triangle between the rivers Euphrates and Tigris-the cradle between pharmacy and civilization. Regulations were in place to preserve public health and hygiene.

The code was first played in recorded history, publicly. Thus, Mesopotamia began man and medicine on the path to civilization – in an unending mission for health and happiness, though the path to happiness was not always flooded with roses [6].

Hippocratic Oath

Hippocrates (460- 377 B.C.) was a Greek physician born in 460 B.C. He became known as the founder of medicine and was regarded as the greatest physician of his time. His medical practice was based on observations and on the study of the human body.

He was recognized as the medicine founder, and was considered the greatest physician of his day. His scientific profession was focused upon findings of human body research. He also correctly identified symptoms of the illness and was the first physician to accurately identify the pneumonia signs. Some of his convictions was trust in the natural healing cycle.

Hippocrates was also the first physician to believe that thoughts, ideas, and feelings come from the brain, and not from the heart, as believed by others of his time. Hippocrates travelled all over Greece practicing his medicine until he reached a medical academy, and then established a Medical Ethics Oath for physicians to observe. Most of the physicians, nowadays, that want to become doctors have to take the Hippocratic Oath as it is in their medical practice. Hippocrates died in 377 BC and today he is known as the "Father of Medicine"

The earliest Greeks believes that disease was punishments sent from the gods. They did not know about the natural causes of diseases and healing until Hippocrates brought that scientific way of thinking. The oath determines the physicist's roles and responsibilities to medicine students and the pupil's roles to trainer. Within the oath the practitioner vows to administer only effective treatments according to his skill and judgment; to refrain from doing pain or injury; and to lead an admirable personal and professional life. Doctors today take the Hippocratic Oath, they swear to be honest, to protect life and to maintain all details confidential between them and patients [4,7].

Moses Maimonides Oath

The Maimonides Oath [8-10] is a cultural oath to pharmacists and doctors attributed to Moses Maimonides (1135-1204), and also attributed to by the acronym Rambam. It is frequently used as the pharmacists' traditional oath, comparable to the Hippocratic Oath to Physicians for which it is also used as a substitute.

The oath; "The eternal providence has appointed me to watch over the life and health of Thy creatures. May the love of my art actuate me at all times; may neither avarice nor miserliness, nor thirst for glory or for a great reputation engage my mind; for the enemies of truth and philanthropy could easily deceive me and make me forgetful of my lofty aim of doing good to Thy children. May I never see in the patient anything but a fellow creature in pain. Grant me the strength, time and opportunity always to correct what I have acquired, always to extend its domain; for knowledge is immense and the spirit of man can extend indefinitely to enrich itself daily with new requirements. Today he can discover his errors of yesterday and tomorrow he can obtain a new light on what he thinks himself sure of today. Oh, God, Thou has appointed me to watch over the life and death of Thy creatures; here am I ready for my vocation and now I turn unto my calling" [8-10].

The Indian Oath

Basic Charaka-samhita text on ancient Indian medicine referred to Charaka, a practitioner of the traditional Indian medicine system known as Ayurveda. Sometime between 2nd century BCE and 2nd century CE Charaka is thought to have prevailed.

It is thought that the Charaka-samhita as it exists today arose in the first Century CE. While Charaka progressed into all aspects of medicine, including the logic and philosophy behind the Indian medicinal system, he put specific focus on disease diagnosis and treated Ayurveda as a comprehensive healthcare system that addressed both preventive and curative aspects. He also explained the classification of different diseases. Ayurvedic medicine is an example of a well-organized system of traditional health care, both preventive and curative, which was broadly accepted in Asian countries. The Charaka Samhita, the biography of Indian Ayurvedic Medicine dating back to around the first century A.D. Instruct physicians "to relieve patients with all your heart and soul; you shall not desert or hurt your patient for your life or life's sake [2, 11].

The English Medical Ethics

In 1772, Thomas Percival (1740 – 1804), a physician of the Manchester Royal Infirmary in England, gathered a comprehensive medical conduct scheme. It was distributed and discussed among his medical colleagues for a decade [12].

The revised dissertation was published in 1803 under the title "Medical Ethics," with two more editions followed. Still a standard work on the topic. Percival advised doctors to "unite tenderness with steadiness, and condescension with authority" to inspire their patients' minds with gratitude, respect and trust [12, 13].

Declaration of Geneva

Adopted by the Second General Assembly of the World Medical Association, Geneva, Switzerland September 1948. It creates on the Hippocratic Oath principles, and is now known as the modern version of it.

It remains one of the WMA's most consistent documents, too. It preserves the ethical values of the medical profession with only a few and cautious revisions over several decades, largely unaffected by contemporary and modernism [14, 15].

Nuremberg Code

In August 1947, following the Nuremberg trials, the Nuremberg Code was implemented. During such courts, Nazi doctors were accused of atrocities committed on concentration camp inmates through human experimentation. It sought to provide specific guidelines for what was and was not legal when human experiments were carried out.

There are 10 points in the code. The first important thing to do is to give informed consent to every participant in an experiment. This means that no one can be forced to take part in human experiments. Everybody needs to consider the possible risks.

The code also provides policies on how to conduct tests. Participants can, for example, leave the experiment if they like. If the doctors know it will hurt the patient, they will stop the experiment. Therefore, there can be no experiment where the risk overweighs the possible benefits [16,17].

Declaration of Helsinki

In order to educate physicians and other scientific research partners including human subjects, the World Medical Association has created the Declaration of Helsinki (by the 18th WMA General Assembly in Helsinki-Finland, June 1964) as a clarification of ethical values. Human scientific work involves studies on human content known or identified data [18].

The Revised Declaration of Geneva

A variety of key ethical standards relating to patient physician interactions, health security, regard for teachers and coworkers among others have been covered by the new version of the Guidelines, and has hence been updated as marginal over the past 70 years since their introduction. A recently updated edition adopted on 14 October 2017 by the WMA General Assembly contains numerous significant changes and improvements (supplement).

The clearest distinction, following references to the Declaration of Geneva, is the clearest acknowledgment of patient rights and other key ethical materials, such as the WMA's Helsinki Declaration: Ethical Principles for Medical Research Concerning Human Subjects and the Taipei Declaration on Ethical Consideration with respect to health data and bio-banks.

With this reason, the working group proposed adding the following guidelines, advised by other members of the WMA, ethics consultants and other experts: "I WILL RESPECT the autonomy and dignity of my patient." Moreover, the Working Group recommended that all new and existing paragraphs on patients' right to the document be changed to include the patient's right of entry, followed by clauses on other professional obligations, to emphasize the importance of patient self-determination as a key cornerstone of medical ethics.

It is expected that the World Medical Association would implement the global Geneva Declaration with this comprehensive review process and follow-up lobbying activities more generally [15,19].

Religion and ethics

One of the well-known facts that religions can show out the very best in people and the very worst, such as marriage and parenthood, like corporations, politics, as well as the industry of healthcare itself. However, these are all institutions that will remain with us and contribute at their best to human prosperity.

Theological contexts gave rise to medicine. The ancients administered their healing oaths to the gods and deities, adding to the task of preserving lives and improving suffering an impression of holy context. The Abrahamic faiths created a revolution in medicine which ultimately led to a more passionate care for the sick than in ancient times. From the Prayer of Maimonides to the establishment of the first Christian hospitals, from the advances of Muslim physicians through the establishment of great medical schools in Europe and the Mediterranean, from the foundation of modern nursing in Florence Nightingale to the setting up of the Hospice movement by Dame Cicely Saunders, from the reverence of life for Albert Schweitzer to liberation theology of Paul Farmer, the noble religious commitment to healing instead energized medical science. There is no inconsistency here, but instead a great collaboration whereby Christian Renaissance humanists such as Francis Bacon establish scientific methods. It means being neglected of its spiritual history that modern medicine is explainable in secular terms. [20].

Successful therapists have often realized that medical art requires patient spirituality to pay empathetic attention. The loved patient feels that in the eyes of the nurse his or her life is worthy and important. The need for meaning, caring love reacts to the deepest needs of humanity. It represents the beloved again, what will otherwise be hidden, meaning, integrity and even value of life. The search for fame or renown is not the need for importance. Rather, everybody needs to feel that their existence is not an error in navigating through life. The recognition of importance in times of serious illness is extremely important [20].

In individuals with serious illnesses spirituality and religion are particularly important. This is a human existence reality — most of those who face a serious threat to their health or the health of a loved one are in their knees and seek help from a more powerful self-understanding. A doctor can be a dedicated atheist, but the average patient does not stop waiting for a major operation to pray for God to guide the surgeon's hands. Many of the surgeons report that patients pray before a major operation and do the best or bow their heads quietly as the patient prays. Spirituality and religion do not "freeze" into the meeting between patient and physician, but are now nothing less constitutive than the early schamanic healers.

Appreciation for patient religious faith should be aligned to respect for physician spirituality in times when a doctor adheres to religious restriction. Principles such as compassion, commitment, diligence and self-improvement are based on the belief in the value of human lives.

How can we improve it? First of all, we should always recognize that religious values are often fundamental to patient identity. Therefore such values cannot be abolished (i.e. left without any effective application in the world within purely the inner dimension of the patient). These values must be considered credible. Secondly, adequately trained clinical spiritual direction should be central to consultations on hospital ethics.

Patients and practitioners also take decisions about health care based about their values and specific religious beliefs. For example, Jehovah's Witnesses generally refuse blood transfusions because it is unaccepted to their religious beliefs, even if such refusal may result in death. A provider of health care may refuse to participate in an abortion because it is against the provider's moral beliefs.

So, medicine and religion are as linked today as they ever were. They are brothers under the skin, for at their best both promote a reverence for life as a gift to be cared for, healed when possible, and freed from physical pain [21].

II. Definition of ethics

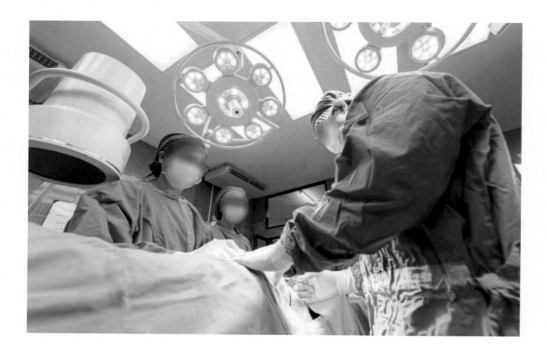

Ethics is the division of philosophy that aims to understand the nature, purposes, justification, and founding principles of moral rules and the systems they compose.

Ethics and morals are descendant from the Greek and Latin terms (roots) for custom. The etymology of the words "ethics" and "morality" is derived from the roots (ethos and mos), which both reflect a meaning describing customs or habits. This etymology supports the anthropologist Ruth Benedict 's claim that all values have their roots in customs and habits of a culture because morality and ethics were essentially developed to describe these subjects [22].

Ethics discusses individual behavior principles. It concentrates on the correctness and error of actions, and the goodness and evil of motives and ends. Ethics involves decision-making in deciding final acts — that is to say, addressing the questions (What should I do?) and (Will it be right?) Ethics represents how people agree to live in accordance with the world and each other across agreed borders and whether they behave in accordance with each other. Ethics, rather than what it really is, is concerned with human behavior as it should be.

Micro-ethics assess the viewpoint for an individual of what is good and wrong, based on the teachings, traditions and experiences of his / her own personal life. Macro-ethics includes a broader understanding of the right and the wrong. Even if nobody lives in vacuum, it does include consideration of ethical issues in a micro and macro perspective to address ethical dilemmas [22].

The term ethics is used in three definite but related ways, signifying

> Philosophical ethics, which involves analysis about ways of life and rules of conduct;
> A general pattern or way of life, such as religious ethics (e.g., Judeo-Christian ethics);
> A set of rules of conduct or "moral code" (e.g., professional codes for ethical behavior).

There are numerous issues in the field of health ethics, including the right to choose or refuse treatment and the right to limit suffering. The process of healthcare decision making has been aggravated by unbelievable technological progress and the resulting capability of extending life beyond what might be seen as a reasonable quality of life.

It is not only about philosophical issues that the scope of healthcare ethics, it's rather covers the economic, healthcare, political, social and legal issues.

Bioethics embraces a wide variety of problems that include the nature of life and death, what kind of life is worth living, how we differentiate between assisted suicide and murder, how we should handle the highly vulnerable persons, and the responsibilities that we have toward other human beings. It aims to make better choices when tackling various complex problems in different circumstances [23,24].

Why We Study Ethics?

We study ethics to assist healthcare providers make wise judgments, good decisions, and right choices; if not right choices, then better choices. To those in the healthcare industry, it is about predicting and recognizing healthcare dilemmas and making sound judgments and decisions based on universal values that work in tandem with the laws of the countries and their constitution.

Where the law remains silent, we depend on the capacity of healthcare givers to make sound judgments, doing the right thing by applying the universal morals and values will help shield and protect all from harm [22].

Ethics deals with:

- ➤ What is right and wrong
- ➤ What is good and bad
- ➤ What ought and ought not to be done.

Medical ethics, therefore, critically examines the reasons that behind any medical decision that involves these concepts. Medical ethics aims to develop and discuss a wise, logical and consistent approach to making moral decisions in medicine [23,24].

It is sometimes helpful to differentiate philosophical medical ethics from law and professional codes of practice, which rely on the interpretation of pre-existing legal and professional rules.

Religious teaching or theological arguments deriving from one or more religious scriptural sources, sociological or psychological reasons why we conduct ourselves in some ways do not necessarily reflect whether the behavior is good or bad. The evaluation of moral decision-making on a historical basis in medicine.

The answer to the question 'What is the right way to do? is not necessarily done. All the disciplines mentioned above can contribute to the medical ethics study [23,24].

Ethical Relativism

The idea of ethical relativism derived by that morality is relative to the standards of the society where one lives. In other words, right or wrong depends on the moral norms of the culture in which it is exercised.

An individual's personal behavior in one community or culture may be legally right and in another it may be incorrect. In one society, what is acceptable cannot be taken for granted in another. Slavery can be regarded an acceptable behavior in one society and unacceptable and inadmissible in another.

The administration of blood may be acceptable as to one's religious beliefs and not acceptable to another within the same community. Patients' legal rights differ between states, as is well known, for example, by Oregon's Death with Dignity Act [25,26].

Healthcare givers need to be aware of social, religious, and legal problems which may influence the extents of what is acceptable and what is unacceptable practice, especially when offering health care to patients with beliefs contrary to their own. The education and training of caregivers become more complicated as different cultures in the world merge into communities. The caregiver not only must understand the clinical skills of his profession but must also be able to understand, both from a legal and an ethical point of view, what is right and what is wrong. Although decision making is not always perfect, the knowledge gained from this practice may assist the health worker in making better decisions [25,26].

The corner stone in medical ethics

Medical ethics is a system of moral principles that apply to practice of clinical medicine and scientific research. It is based on certain principles, some make it four basic principles, and other consider five points or six points, or even seven points. The English philosopher W D Ross, used the term "prima facie" which means the principle binding unless its conflicts with another moral principles, if it does, we have to choose between them [27,28,29].

Those principles do not provide order or rules, but can help doctors and other health care providers to make decision when reflecting on moral issues that arise on work.

The four principles are [27-30]:

1. Respect for autonomy

The principle of autonomy involves admitting the right of a person to make one's own decisions. "Auto" comes from a Greek word meaning "self" or the "individual." Autonomy- literally, self-rule, but may be better described as considered self-rule is a special attention to all moral aspects. In other words, it means recognizing an individual's right to make his or her own decisions about what is best for him- or herself. So the patient has the right to accept or to reject the recommended plan for management. If the patient has the power autonomy, he can make his decision on the bases of consultation.

The principle of autonomy is not absolute. One person's autonomous actions must not violate another's rights. All people deserve the right to make their own healthcare choices. A patient has the right to reject healthcare, even if it helps to save his or her life. Patients may refuse treatment, refuse medication and refuse invasive procedures irrespective of their benefits. They have a right to manage their decisions adhered to by family members who may disagree simply because they are unable to let go. Although patients have a right to make their own choices, they also have a complimentary right to know the risks, benefits, and alternatives to recommended procedures.

What happens when the right to autonomy conflicts with other moral principles, such as beneficence and justice? Conflict can arise, for example, when a patient refuses a blood transfusion considered necessary to save his or her life while the caregiver's primary requirement is to do no harm. Determining the right thing to do in any given situation is not always an easy decision [31].

Medical confidentiality is another meaning of respecting patient autonomy. Maintaining confidentiality not only respecting patients' autonomy but also improves the chances of our being capable to help them.

2. Beneficence

Beneficence describes the principle of a well doing, this reflects to produce the benefit to patient with no harm, and expressing kindness, showing compassion, and helping others. In the healthcare setting, workers have to demonstrate beneficence by providing benefits and balancing benefits against risks. Beneficence requires one to do good. Certainly whenever we try to help others, we inevitably risk harm to them but the harm should be minimized to the least possible.

Strict and successful preparation and education must be provided for this purpose. Doing good needs to be well informed of the beliefs, culture, values, and preferences of the patient, what one individual may believe to be good for a patient may in reality be harmful. For example, a caregiver may decide to tell a patient frankly, "There is nothing else that I can do for you." This may be harmful to the patient if the patient truly asks encouragement and information about care options from the caregiver.

Compassion here allows the healthcare giver tell the patient to say: "I am not aware of modern treatments of your condition, but I have some thoughts about how I can improve it, to make it more convenient to treat your symptoms. I will also keep you informed of any major research which can be useful in dealing with your disease processes".

Sadly some surgical procedures in one end produce benefit but on the other end produce harm to the body or even to the psyche, but this is inevitable.

3. Non Maleficence

Non-maleficence is an ethical principle that requires caregivers to avoid causing patients harm. It derives from the ancient maxim (primum non nocere), translated from the Latin, "first, do no harm." Physicians nowadays still swear by the code of Hippocrates, promising to do no harm. This means no harm to be done to the patient under any condition and for any reason, we have to watch when we can offer to the patients if we feel we cannot do good then we should not do harm. Medical ethics requires healthcare providers to "first, do no harm." A New Jersey court in In re Conroy18 found that "the physician's primary obligation is . . . First do no harm."

Telling the truth, for example, can sometimes cause harm. If there is no cure for a patient's disease, you may face a conflict. Do I tell the patient and possibly cause serious psychological harm, or do I give the patient what I consider to be false hopes? Is there a middle ground? If so, what is it? To avoid causing harm, alternatives may need to be considered in solving the ethical dilemma.

The caregiver, realizing that he or she cannot help a particular patient, attempts to avoid harming the patient. This is done as a caution against taking a serious risk with the patient or doing something that has no immediate or long-term benefits [33].

4. Justice (equality in offering treatment)

Often regarded as being synonymous with fairness. Can be defined as moral obligation to act on the basis of fair adjunction between competing claims. Justice in medical is fair distribution of scarce resources (distributive justice). We think that adding respect to patient's dignity is necessary, will be five instead of four.

Some writers count it as six in the following way, beneficence, non-maleficence, respect for autonomy, justice, dignity, and truthfulness/honesty.

Another writers consider the code as:

Respect for autonomy, fidelity, justice, beneficence, non-maleficence, veracity and deontological.

Double effect is noticed sometimes in medical practice, which mean serving the patient in one direction, but in the same time producing harm like prescribing morphine to relieve pain and suffering.

Other principles of ethics

Ethical principles are universal rules of conduct, based on ethical theories which provide a practical basis for determining what kinds of actions, intentions, and motives are valued. Ethical principles help caregivers to make choices according to moral principles which have been specified as standards considered meaningful when addressing health care–related ethical conflicts. As noted by the principles discussed in the following sections, caregivers, in the study of ethics, will find that difficult decisions often involve choices between conflicting ethical principles.

Response for human rights

The era of human rights began with the formation of the UN, which promoted human rights in 1945.

The first text that established human rights was the Universal Declaration of Human Rights (1948).

Medical doctors had an ethical responsibility to defend the rights of patients and their human dignity, which has had an effect on medical ethics through the advent of the document define human rights.

Referral

Physicians who earn interests from referring patients to medical test or imaging have been found to refer more [34]. The practice is prohibit by the American College

Of Physician Ethics Manual [35]. Fee splitting and the payments of promotions to recruit several of patients is explained unethical and unacceptable all over the world.

Confidentiality

Confidentiality is usually referred to conversations between physician and patients, this principle is comment soon as patient-physician privilege. Legal protection prohibit doctors from displaying their conversation with patients even under Oath in the court [36].

Vendor relationship

Studies shows that physician can be motivated by drug or instruments companies, including gifts like trips, dinners, and congress fees [37]. Industry-sponsored Continuous Medical Education program affects prescribing pattern. So it is much better to stop this industry support, as some American universities have banned pharmaceutical industry-sponsored gifts and royalties.

Futility

Medical futility referred to interventions which are uncertain to give any considerable benefit for the patient [38]. This is ethical and religious conflict, deception is not accepted any way. Sometimes the court obligate offering treatment, this situations are faced with terminally ill patients and in children with severe congenital anomalies, in the Islamic law the doctor have to support his patient till the last moment of his life.

Paternalism

Paternalism is a form of beneficence. Sometimes people believe that they know what is best for someone else and take decisions that they believe are in the best interest of that person. It could include, for example, retaining data, believing that the patient would be better off that way. Paternalism may occur because of one's age, cognitive ability, and level of dependency.

When a third party imposes its wishes on others, the right of a patient to self-determination is compromised.

Medical paternalism usually related to physicians which inadvertently making decisions for patients who are capable of making their own choices. Physicians often find themselves in situations where they can manipulate a patient's healthcare decision simply by selectively telling the patient what he or she prefers based on their own beliefs. This actively breaches the patient autonomy.

The problem of paternalism involves a conflict between the principles of autonomy and beneficence, each of which may be viewed and expressed differently, for example, by the physician and patient, physician and family member, or even the patient and a family member.

Ultimately, as determined by court decisions, it is the patient's right to know and choose what line of management they wish to pursue without undue pressure from the physician [39].

Pillars of Moral Strength

There is an enumerate number of ethical issues in every side of human existence. In spite of the cultural differences, politics, and religion, that impact who we are, it is all of our life experiences that influence who we have become. If we have courage to do right, those who have influenced our lives were most likely courageous. If we are compassionate, it is presumably because we have been influenced by the compassionate.

The pillars of moral strength depicts a virtuous human. What is it that distinguishes every human apart? In the final analysis, it is the person's virtues and values that build moral character. Look beyond the words and ask, "Do I know their meanings?" "Do I apply their concepts?" "Do I know their value?" "Are they part of me?" [22].

Empathy and compassion

Empathy and compassion are offer a lot for the process of healing, but evidence suggests a deterioration during the exercise and real life practice. Compassion means recognition, understanding, emotional response, empathy for other people's concerns, struggling, sadness, pain and suffering, and recognition, motivation and relational action to improve those conditions.

Beth A Lown [40] assumed that, neuroscientists have recognized neural networks that generate shared representations of directly experienced and observed feelings, sensations and actions. When shared representations stimulate empathic concern or compassion for another's painful situation, humans experience compassionate motivation to help. The resulting attitude are affected with activation of areas in the brain associated with conjunction and reward.

Activation of these neural networks is sensitive to a lot of inter- and intra-personal motivations. These include the ability to concentrate person's attention, the ability to obtain and accurately assess input about distress, the perception one adopts in order to understand another's experience, self-other boundary awareness, the extent to which one values another's welfare, the ability to understand and regulate one's own emotions, the skills to attend to one's own wellbeing through self-care and self-compassion, impressive communication skills, reflection and meta-cognition.

His research conclusion suggests that compassion can be influenced by education and training and is linked with positive emotions, a sense of affiliation, reward and pro-social behaviors. A compassion process design and structure with examples of educational goals, interventions and resources for curriculum development are described. However, education must be continuous with changes in clinical practice to sustain compassionate care.

Detachment

Detachment, or lack of concern for the patient's needs, often converts into mistakes that result in patient harm. Those who have extreme emotional involvement in a patient's care should be most suitable for working in those settings where patients are most likely to recover and have good outcomes (e.g., maternity units). As with all things in life, there needs to be a comfortable balance between compassion and detachment [22,41].

III. Patient Rights and Responsibilities

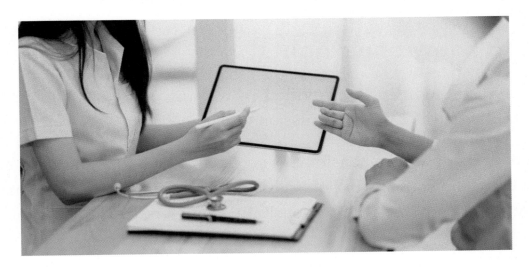

Aprofessional relationship between the physician and the patient is vital for the administration of proper medical care. The medical staff and the patients must be aware of and understand not only their own rights and responsibilities but also the rights and responsibilities of one another [42].

Patient rights

The continuing raise of consumer awareness, linked with increased governmental regulations, makes it prudent for caregivers to recognize the scope of patient rights.

Confirming that the rights of patients are secured, needs more than educating policy makers and health providers; it requires educating individuals about the kind of treatment and respect to which they should expect from their governments and their health care providers. People will then play a significant role in raising the quality of treatment if their own expectation standards are increased [43-46].

Right to know one's rights

Patients have a right to be provided in writing a copy of their rights and responsibilities at the time of admission to the hospital.

The patient's rights and responsibilities are documented in a statement most often referred to as The Patient's Bill of Rights. The general public should have access to a copy of patient rights and responsibilities upon request [43-46].

Right to explanation of one's rights

Patients have a right to receive an explanation of their rights and responsibilities. The rights of patients must be respected at all times. Each patient is an individual with unique healthcare needs. The patient has a right to make decisions regarding his or her medical care, including the decision to discontinue treatment, to the extent permitted by law [43-46].

Right to ask questions

The patient has a right to ask questions and caregivers have a responsibility to listen. Caregivers should not become dismissive or minimize the value of a patient's opinion as to the cause of his or her medical complaints and conditions. Even if a patient may be anxious, the questions asked must not be disregarded.

Patients have the right to ask questions regarding their care from entry to the hospital through the time of departure. Questions regarding care should include, for example, "I saw blood in my IV tubing. Is this okay? Is it infiltrating?" or "My wound dressing seems wet. Is this okay? Should the dressing be changed?"

Patients should not hesitate to ask for [43-46]:

> ➤ Explanation of a caregiver's instructions
> ➤ Interpretation of a caregiver's handwriting
> ➤ Instructions for medication usage (e.g., frequency, dosing, drug–drug or drug–food interactions, contraindications, side effects)
> ➤ Verification of a physician's diet orders
> ➤ Clarification of the treatment plan
> ➤ A copy of the organization's hand washing policy
> ➤ A description of the hospital's instructions to prevent wrong-site surgery
> ➤ Consultations and second opinions
> ➤ Precise and complete discharge instructions
> ➤ Verification that their advance directives are on file (e.g., living will)
> ➤ Confirmation that contact information for the patient's alternate decision maker is on file in case that the patient becomes incapacitated and cannot make healthcare decisions [47].

Right to complain

Patients have a right to file a complaint when they are dissatisfied with their care and treatment.

Right to emergency care

Emergency care is well recognized as a patient right.

Right to admission

In case the patient is designated to admission to a specific hospital depends on the judgment establishing that hospital. Governmental hospitals, for example, are by definition organizations of some unit of government; their principle concern is to provide service to the population within the administration of that unit.

Right to examination and treatment

Patients have a right to consider the physician will make a relevant history and physical examination based to the patient's presenting complaints. The assessment is the method by which a physician evaluate the patient's condition of health, looking for signs of trauma and disease. It offer's the base for a specifically evaluating the patient's health problems, which leads to successful recovery strategy upon treatment plan. A careless assessment may end with misdiagnosis and inappropriate treatment plan.

As reported by Karen Asp in Shape Magazine, "It took almost my whole life to get the right diagnosis because no one person had asked me enough questions" [48].

Right to know caregivers

Patients basically, have a right to enquire the names and positions of the health care workers who will care for them while in the hospital. Patients should know who is treating them by name, discipline, role, and responsibility in their care plan. Caregivers should identify themselves to patients by name and discipline.

Right to informed consent

Patients have a right to obtain a thorough explanation of treatment modalities which helps to make an informed decision prior to consenting to a predetermined procedure or treatment. The physician has responsibility to provide the patient informed consent that includes the risks, benefits, and alternatives of each procedure or treatment option. The right to obtain information from the physician includes knowledge about the disease, the suggested line of management, and the prospects of recovery in a language that is very clear to the patient.

The physician must honestly balance the risks and benefits of each treatment method. This balancing act may lead to a conflict where the physician's recommended procedure differs from the procedure the patient is willing to accept. Pressing a patient to undergo an unwanted procedure is a form of paternalism which may reflect a failure to respect the patient's right of self-determination [43-46].

Right to refuse treatment

It's the responsibility of the patient for his actions if he refuses treatment or do not follow the practitioner's instructions, as far as he is capable to make decision.

For the patient who leaves against medical advice, it's better to follow the framework "assess, investigate, mitigate, explain, and document." [49,50].

Right to execute advance directives

Patients have the right to eliminate advance directives. A patient who becomes incapacitated or unable to make decisions on his or her own behalf has a right to assign a stand-in decision maker to make decisions on his or her behalf [43-46].

Right to have special needs addressed

Patients who have language barriers or hearing or vision impairments have a right to specific aid to make their needs addressed in order to enhance the quality of care. Many healthcare organizations maintain a list of employees with various language skills and sign-language expertise in order to provide patients with high-quality care [43-46].

Right to Choose Physician(s)

Generally, patients have a right to choose their treating physician. However, in urgent and emergent cases, there may be no time to identify the physician of choice because of life-threatening injuries, such as may occur in an automobile accident. In an elective surgical case, for example, after choosing a surgeon, the patient has the right to expect that the chosen operating surgeon will really perform such surgery to which the patient has consented [43-46]. In case that after signing a consent form, the patient was operated on by another surgeon in the same field, even when the two surgeons are engaged in a group practice, it's considered as malpractice. Some courts where that another surgeon operate on one's patient without the patient's knowledge and consent considers as deceit [51].

Right to trust caregivers

Trust is a vital issue for patients that can be used as an indicator and potential 'marker' for how patients assess the quality of health care.

The critical aspect that trust roles in qualified doctor–patient relationships has been well understood. Trust has been proven to be a vital issue affecting a wide range of important therapeutic plans including patient acceptance of therapeutic recommendations, adherence to recommendations, satisfaction with recommendations, satisfaction with medical care, symptom improvement and patient disenrollment [52].

Right to patient advocacy services

Joint Commission standards state that the "patient has the right to access protective and advocacy services." Most organizations have approved guideline and programs to address patient complaints. A patient generally understands patient concerns.

Access to a patient advocate is mostly explained in patient's handbooks. Patient advocacy services have to be feasible to both patients and families [53].

Right to have spiritual needs assessed and addressed

Patients are able to chaplaincy assistance and to determine and meet their religious beliefs. The aim of a system of pastoral care is to reinforce the essential function performed by spiritual care as a part of the healing cycle of the patient. The program would also offer emotional guidance to patients and their family in compliance with their desires when they are in the facility. The hospital supports the position of pastors and participants in religious education as critical health care professionals.

Many hospitals provide a multi-religious center as well as TV coverage. Many hospitals offering regular spiritual commitment and contemplation. Music and meditation are also given as a complement to the relaxation of pain and tension on the bedside [54,55].

Right to ethics consultation

The privileges of patients in certain hospitals require patients and/or relatives to contact an ethics committee in the case of challenging medical decisions including ethical dilemmas. Conflicts are also produced when a detrimental outcome happens in two or more choices. Controversy will occur because the opinion of families and caregivers vary or when the family is uncertain about the appropriate method of handling the individual. Consultation of the Ethics Committee can provide an objective view. Ethics committees are consultative in nature.

Ethics Committee advice should not be regarded as enforceable. Consultations on ethics are beneficial when taking final decisions, like end-of-life decisions [56].

Right to choose treatment

Patients should be able to choose the medical treatment they want. They have the right to know and accept or deny care of their therapeutic approaches. The more advanced medical technology, the more difficult care decisions are to take. Should I have the surgery? Do I need to be maintained on a ventilator? Usually, these decisions constitute not only medical questions but moral and ethical conflict as well. What has the greater value, the length of life or the quality of life? What is the right choice? Although patients have a right to make their own care and treatment decisions, they often face conflicting religious and moral values in their decision-making process. Often, it is hard to make a choice when two roads may seem equally desirable [57,58].

Right to respect

The right to respect is a common right retained by patients, families, and caregivers. Respect is more than a two-way street. It is not just about what is right for you and me rather it promotes respect of all persons irrelevant to culture and religious beliefs [58].

Right to pain management

Pain is the method of the body for warning the patient that something is not very good. Pain management is the procedure by which caregivers act with the patient to assess the pain generator and create a pain control treatment plan. The procedure includes educating the patient as to the value of pain management in the healing process. With modern medications, mostly the pain can be prevented or at least be better controlled.

Patients have a right to have a pain evaluation and treatment of any established pain. A pain rating scale is a visual tool usually used to help patients describe the level of pain. It assists the healthcare worker to know how good medications are working and if a change in the treatment plan is necessary. The pain assessment scale is a tool usually used because of its simplicity of use in achieving the goal. As much important as the severity of pain are its locations and type (e.g., burning sensation, throbbing, dull, stabbing, numbing, sharp, shooting). A diagram of the body could be helpful so the patient can more easily points the various locations of his or her pain. The severity of pain can be described to the physician to assist in diagnosing and treating the patient. All patients have a right to [43-46]:

> A pain control management plan specified with the help of the caregiver
> Alternative and/or complementary procedures included in the pain management plan that might help improve the efficacy of traditional treatment options (e.g., pain medications), for example, acupuncture, imagery, meditation, reiki (ancient Japanese touch therapy)
> Inclusion of family and caregivers in the decision-making process

➢ Explanation of the medications, anesthesia, or other treatments planned
➢ An explanation of the risks, benefits, and alternatives (e.g., acupuncture) to suggested treatment(s)
➢ Request changes in treatment if pain persists
➢ Refuse pain treatment(s), even if they were recommended
➢ Receive pain medication in a timely manner

Patient responsibilities

Patients also have the conditions to hold on certain obligations. The hospital defines these responsibilities and then transfer them to the patient. When patients understand and accept their responsibilities, the concept of the patient as a partner in care becomes a dynamic aspect of the patient's episode of care [59-61].

Maintain a healthy lifestyle

Living a healthy lifestyle involves both a right and a responsibility. Every individual have to take responsibility for living well through exercise, diet, stress control, and maintaining positive social relationships, which will be validated with a richer and fuller life hoping that its better prepare people for whatever health obstacles the future may face. Realizing what is right and what is wrong for one's health is not enough; it must be recognized and practiced [59-61].

Keep appointments

Patients bears the obligation for a timely announce the caregivers whenever they are not capable to keep the scheduled appointment. Failure to alarm caregivers of appointment withdrawal leads to longer delays for other patients, which cannot be easy to re-arrange appointments with physicians.

Maintain current medication records

Patients must keep always an updated precise record of their drugs, including dosages, route of administration, and frequency. Drug allergies have be mentioned (if any). Medication records should be reviewed regularly to be sure the listing remains up to date. A list should be given to treating physicians and treating facility.

Accurately Describe Symptoms

Patients have a responsibility to precisely describe symptoms, family history, the location and severity of pain.

Provide Full and Honest Disclosure of Medical History

Patients have a concern to fully disclose of all information pertaining to his\her medical condition, medical complaints, symptoms, location and severity of pain, previous pain control issues, past illnesses, treatments, surgical or other invasive procedures, hospitalizations, medications, and allergies. Information delivered should be precise, valid, and complete.

The selectivity of the information delivered to the treating doctor or healthcare center for whatever the cause will lead caregivers down the wrong way when managing the case [59-61]. Reasons for that, in some patients they feel that's embarrassing to tell information, like loss of sphincter control, sex life or domestic violence, other reason that the patient aware from blaming, judging or lecturing doctor, if the patient tell him the truth that he was not stick to the treatment plan, taking unhealthy diet, or exercise [62,63].

Adhere to the treatment plan

Patient noncompliance has been recognized as a global public health concern which puts a major financial burden upon current health care services. There is comprehensive literature into the definition, assessment and treatment of patient's non-compliance. Nevertheless, one-third to half of patients refuse to comply with professional recommendations and medications.

When the patient refuses to follow the treatment plan of a physician, the caregiver will be disappointed. The duty of proper consideration lies with both the caregiver, in relating to the patient the importance of complying with the treatment plan, and the patient, who has the obligation to obey the physician's recommendations. Ultimately, patient care outcomes will progress when patients comply with their prescribed management strategies. Healthcare providers really do have to consider and discuss the issue of patient's noncompliance in designing care strategies. For seniors with cognitive disabilities, this is particularly relevant [64].

Follow discharge instructions

Patients are not necessarily consistent when following the discharge instructions of the physician and/or hospital. It's better for both the hospitals and physicians to have a follow-up process for their patients. The process must contain a documented discharge plan that is signed by the patient, who have to be provided with a copy of it [59-61].

IV. Informed Consent

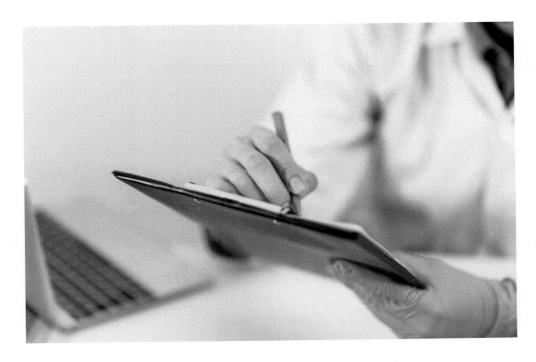

Informed consent is a top priority because it protects both patients and doctors. It's a safety valve for the health care providers if performed perfect, and up to the required level.

It's very vital to be sure that the patient understands the health care provider language clearly. Also, the doctor should evaluate the patients' capability to have the mental ability to sign.

Some patients, like children, mentally retarded, and patients with dementia or psychological disturbance, are not capable of even understanding the details to sign. In that case, someone else (proxy), will sign on their benefit.

Informed consent should be prepared before any procedure, no matter how minor or major it is. It's better to be performed in a private and quite room. The doctor should make himself totally free at this time. The patient has the right to have escort during this discussion.

Fine communication skills are required with a warm welcoming, and a big smile. The treating doctor can do this by initiating conversation, asking questions and communicating clearly [65].

The following points are required to be clarified to the patients.

> Careful description of the patients' diagnosis and treatment.
> Allow for open questions.
> To clarify some points, videos or pictures may be required.
> Every point must be documented in the patients' chart.
> Careful listening to the patients' remarks, questions, and careful observation for the patients' body language.
> Ask for the feedback, and ask the patient to tell what he understood from the message given.
> If the patient is having a serious condition, gentleness is required to clarify the situation.
> Avoid medical jargon when describing the treatments.
> Beware of religious and cultural differences, which may affect understanding.

➢ Requite an interpreter if necessary.

All options must be described

Treating physician should totally warn the patient of the risks and benefits of each procedure prior to undertake the intervention. The explanation must be in a language that the patient understands and include full information regarding alternative treatments. The patient cannot make an informed choice for one treatment if he/she does not know of the existence of others.

All major adverse effects must be described

Adverse effects and harm from medical care do not necessarily reflect a mistake or failure of therapy. The error was if not informing the patient of an alternative option in management. At the same time, a patient could potentially die as an adverse effect of treatment. This is only an ethical and legal issue when the adverse event occurs and the patient was not told that it may have happened. The patient might say, "Doctor, I would never have taken pregabalin, if you had told me it might cause a blurred vision, constipation, or fatigue" or "I would never have had surgery if you had told me I might need a blood transfusion." The main point is to respect patient's autonomy. The patients should be warned of the therapeutic options, the adverse effects of the procedure, and the harm of not undergoing the procedure. If they have the ability to recognize and they choose to do it anyway, they have made an autonomous therapeutic choice, and accordingly, the patient holds the burden of any adverse effect, not the physician.

The patient have to understand the risks of the intervention just like a driver must understand the risks before getting behind the steering wheel of a car. Why can't accuse a car manufacturer if people die in a car accident? Predominantly because they are mature with the capacity to understand the risks of driving and they chose to drive anyway.

In addition to understanding the risks of the procedure, treating doctor must inform the patient of what could happen if he or she does not choose therapy that you offer.

For example, a patient comes to the emergency department with cauda equina syndrome, because of herniated disc in the lumbar spine. He is informed of the risks of surgery, and refuses the procedure both verbally and in writing. Then, the patient ends with a permanent neural deficit. What was done wrong here?

The patients must be informed both of the risk of the treatment, as well as, what will happen if they don't undergo the procedure. In this case the physician is liable in court if he never documented that he informed the patient of the possibility of permanent neurological deficit if the patient did NOT have the procedure [66].

Consent is required for each specific procedure

If the patient signs a consent form for an operation on her left knee, you cannot, in the operating room, decide to operate on her right knee and assume that you have consent. If a patient signs a consent for a herniated disc prolapse in a certain level, but when you open her up you find signs of instability you cannot just do the spinal fixation without prior informing the patient and family of the additional procedure and obtaining their consent. There can be no presumption for consent for anything beyond what the patient specifically said he\she consented to. Either the patients have to sign consent in advance for the other procedures or they have to regain consciousness and have the additional procedure explained to them [66].

Beneficence not sufficient to eliminate the need for consent

Trying to be sincere and to do well is highly important and takes primacy; however, the patient's right to control what happens with his own body is more important. This is true even if the intervention will save the patient's life, unless the illness is an emergency in an unconscious patient.

Beneficence does not minimize the need for informed consent. If you live in a very messy place your neighbor cannot break into your room to clean it even if he doesn't steal anything. You must consent to the cleaning. His good intentions are not as significant as your right to do what you want with your own property [66].

V. Ethics in Patient Assessments and Diagnosis

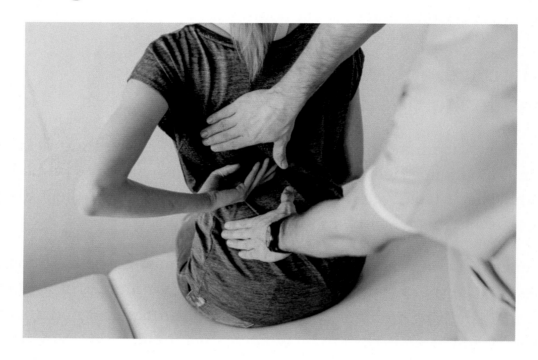

Patient evaluation involves the systematic gathering and interpreting of patient-specific data necessary to help identify a patient diagnosis, from which base the patient's care and treatment strategies. The patient's method of care is only as successful as evaluations operated by the experts of the various disciplines (e.g., physicians, nurses, dietitians, physical therapists).

The physician's evaluation involves a review of the patient's history, symptoms, and physical examination results. This needs to be performed within 24 hours of a patient's admission to the hospital. The findings of the clinical examination are used to configure the patient's plan of care. A superficial and lazy evaluation will lead to a misdiagnosis of the patient's health struggles and/or proper care needs and, subsequently, to poor care.

It is doubtful in some cases as to whether a healthcare worker actually completes the process of obtaining a patient's medical history when he\she simply draws a diagonal line from the top right to the bottom left of the form and writes through the line "unremarkable".

Failure to obtain a proper medical history and physical examination breaches the standard of care owed to the patient [67].

Wisdom in using investigations

Patient diagnosis may, in addition to the history and examination, needs screen tests, and the results of investigations such as ECG, imaging studies, and laboratory tests findings that assists health care providers to reach the final diagnosis and define the treatment plan.

An impressive fact is that when hands-on doctoring fades away, patients lose. In some hospitals today, the average amount of time a busy intern spends with a patient is four minutes. No longer are tests ordered based on the results of a careful history and physical examination, but what is more worse is the dependence on the technology without touching the patient as technological investigations become the primary input of information on the patients. This behavior should be stopped, because this process is driving up health-care costs posed by sometimes unnecessary and risky procedures [68].

Even with all the diagnostic utilities available to physicians, if they order the tests and fail to review or interpret them in accordance with a patient's physical complaints and medical history, they are of little or no value. Tests results from imaging studies (like MRI) are useless in arriving at an accurate diagnosis and appropriate treatment plan if they are merely filed away after a cursory review [67].

Medications

With thousands of brand-name and generic drugs in use, it is no surprise that drug errors are one of the leading causes of patient injuries. Physicians should encourage the limited and judicious use of all medications and should document periodically the reason for their continuation. They should be alert to any contraindications and incompatibilities among prescription and over-the-counter drugs, and herbal supplements. Medication errors often occur due to administration of the wrong medication to the wrong patient of the wrong dosage at the wrong site by the wrong route, or a combination of all these.

Another important issue here, is narcotic drugs, specially for patients with chronic low back pain, post-surgical patients, or patients with failed back surgery syndrome, and in addition to all is the psychological factor. Here, the treating doctor should be very cautious in prescribing narcotics, and closely observe the patient for any behavioral change, to identify misuse and document the specific aberrant behaviors for reference. Such documentation justifies doctors' decision not to prescribe harmful substances. But before everything, we should never abandon the patient in pain, rather than to look for the real pain generator ant treat it radically [69,70].

Patient-Doctor relationship

The relationship between patients and doctors is at the core of medical ethics, serving as an anchor for many of the most important debates in the field.

The patient-doctor relationship entails special obligations for the physician to provide care to his or her patient. The physician's principle responsibility should always be the patient's benefit and best interests, whether the physician is preventing or treating illness or helping the patient to cope with disease, disability, and death. It has well been observed that the health and interest of the patient based on a harmonious action between the doctor and the patient. The doctor should support the dignity of all patients and respect their individualism [71,72].

During the past several decades, this relationship has evolved along three interrelated axes — as it is defined in clinical care, research, and society.

The patient-doctor relationship in the clinical realm has historically been framed in terms of beneficial paternalism. Until about 1960, most codes of medical ethics based mainly on the Hippocratic tradition, framing the obligations of physicians firmly in terms of advancing the benefits of the patient, while keeping silent about patients' rights. In the following years basic cultural changes have contributed to an expansion in individual resistance toward governmental and institutional control, a growth in rights-based protests, with patient rights rising as common norm as well as the rights of protections for women, ethnic groups' rights, minority rights and others.

This abrupt transition shifts the authority in decision making from the treating doctor to the patient. And moreover, with the development of the Internet, its countless websites related to health and other sources of medical information, many patients felt that they are largely able to manage their own medical conditions and that doctors are mainly consultants. Nevertheless, the reality is more complex: the abundance of medical knowledge available to patients has proved to be as harmful as it is helpful, and today patients and physicians are starting to achieve a healthier balance of authority through an approach of shared decision making. With this process, doctors are seen as sharing expertise and authority over issues of medical science, whereas patients' main concerns over questions of principles and priorities.

This separation of work represents a recognition of the pragmatic deception, the mistaken belief that physician can acquire ethical conclusions from scientific facts; actually, an "ought" should not be deduced from an "is." Even when clinicians should provide experience in the medical knowledge of a patient's condition, such findings are never enough to determine the line of management. Clinical decisions should therefore take into account the patient's beliefs and preferences.

This strategy has many ramifications; for example, in understanding the ability of a competent adult to deny a lifesaving blood transfusion depending on his or her religious values, or the freedom of a patient to reject mechanical ventilation for a treatable and reversible cause of respiratory failure. In other terms the patient should come before the system.

More important, however, is the method that the approach of shared decision making leads the many more banal decisions that are made in clinics every day, when clinicians provide patients with what they see as reasonable medical options and then help them to merge personal values and preferences to reach at decisions that make the most reasonable for them in terms of both the medical realities and their unique individual perspective. This strategy of engaging patients has more benefits as well, like promoting their sense of self-efficacy and improving their adherence to treatment instructions [71,73].

Patient-Reported Outcome

Analyzing relevant outcomes in a regular bases is a primary concern in a health care system largely concentrated on the provision of high-value care. Most quality assessments concentrates on care processes or downstream outcomes such as survival; until recently, there has been less motivation on quantitative measurements of functional outcomes, symptoms, and quality of life [74].

Measuring patient-reported outcomes (PROs) with standardized questionnaires is a method of obtaining this information. PRO collection has abounded in oncology, where it has been connected to improved symptom management, improved quality of life, and longer survival [75].

Given these merits, payers have started to advance healthcare providers to merge PRO collection into routine care. Some institutions includes financial incentives for hospitals to collect and submit PRO data for patients undergoing elective surgeries.

Other institutions have incorporated PRO collection into daily practice and have seen promising results [76].

Nevertheless, despite familiarity with PROs has grown, feedback has progressively underscored that clinicians find organizing PROs to be beneficial rather than exhausted. Information from qualified consumers shows that PRO selection is not only practical and beneficial for healthcare services, but also for other purposes may improve physician efficiency and reduce burnout, for many reasons:

First, PROs will enhance patient-doctor relationship by enabling healthcare providers to adequately understand patients' symptoms. For instance, the set PROs provided spine surgeons a quantitative estimation of the level to which patients were suffering to handle with their postsurgical pain. Surgeons may then take appropriate steps, like transferring specific patients to a behavioral pain psychologist. PROs also provided suppliers a more data derived from interpretation of post-procedure recovery profiles. The information obtained from these evaluations usually varies from physicians' long-standing concepts and assisted them better combine with patients throughout the recovery process.

Moreover PROs may improve combined decision making. For example, if a surgeon described an elderly patient who insisted on having a radical excision with safe margin for a sacral chordoma, during abstract discussions about incontinence, impotence, and other possible neural injuries proved unpersuasive, but when showing him real patient data on post-operative over time catalyzed a conversation about risks and benefits that led to the patient's choosing marginal excision and radiation therapy. Both the physician and the patient felt better about the process and outcome of their PRO-facilitated conversation.

Second, and most surprisingly, PROs may improve workflow efficiency and save time when they're used regularly. One primary care physician noted that using electronic surveys that included a screening questionnaire, risk assessments, and a review of systems enabled her to improve her bedside practice. Because patients had already answered screening questions electronically while in her clinic's waiting room, she was no longer obligated to pass through verbal checklists during visits.

Finally, PROs have encouraged conversations that might not otherwise have taken place by allowing sensitive problems to be discussed in systematic manner. Radiation oncologists reported that PROs have enabled honest conversations related to sexual dysfunction, incontinence, and rectal bleeding in patients with prostate cancer [77].

Thus, our suggestion is that the use of PROs can improve physician satisfaction, enhance physician–patient relationships, increase workflow efficiency, and enable crucial conversations.

Increasing physician satisfaction is vital given that almost half of physicians have at least one symptom of burnout, and burnout is associated with medical errors, lower patient satisfaction, and decreased patient compliance to treatment plans [78,79].

Breaking bad news to patients

Breaking bad news is among of the most daunting procedures that healthcare workers have to accomplish in every day practice. For many, their first practice involves patients they have known only a short time. Moreover, they are required upon to break the bad news with little planning or training. Given the integral nature of bad news, which is, the news that dramatically and negatively impacts the patient's view of her or his life, this is hardly a formula for success.

Bad news is defined as any information that adversely and negatively affects the patients' view of future. When a patient receives bad news, his/her life changes. The way such information are provided is highly critical because the shortage of satisfactory experience and knowledge will inversely affect both the patient and physician. Physicians consider this process complex and stressful. Delivering bad news has psychological impacts on both patient and doctor. Studies have shown that patients have the need and interest to know the truth. So, when they think that their doctor is not sincere, it makes them more worried and destroys their trust [80].

Historically, physicians protected patients from bad news. Hippocrates recommended "concealing most things from the patient," as many "have taken a turn for the worse ... by forecast of what is to come." In the original Code of Ethics, the American Medical Association reiterated this belief and advised physicians to "avoid all things which have a tendency to discourage the patient." This concept continued through the mid-20th century when studies showed that most doctors would avoid disclosing a cancer unless specifically requested.

While the principle of non-maleficence likely promoted this approach, modification for nondisclosure depends on two key assumptions: the first is that the patients do not want the truth, or second is the patients cannot handle the truth. However, these suggestions have never been confirmed. In contrary, patient evaluations have revealed that they would prefer to be informed the reality for a difficult diagnosis. Shielding information may exacerbate confusion or delay treatment and is usually detrimental [81].

Furthermore, medical education have been granted higher emphases on technical proficiency than communication skills. This makes physicians not very well prepared for the communication complexity and emotional intensity of delivering bad news. The worries physicians have about breaking bad news include; fears of being blamed, triggering a bad reaction, expressing emotion, not knowing all the answers, worries of the unknown and untaught, and personal fear of illness and death. This will make doctors to become emotionally unengaged from their patients. Moreover, bad news delivered inadequately or insensitively will deteriorate patients' and relatives' long-term adjustments to the consequences of that news.

The best exercise which adopt a patient-centered approach that includes the patient's family. A patient- and family-centered approach not only maintain the patient at the center, but has also been shown to express the highest patient satisfaction and results in the physician being recognized as emotional, available, expressive of hope, and not dominant.

In a patient- and family-centered program, the doctor reveals the information according to the patient's and patient's family's needs. Specifying these needs takes in consideration the cultural, spiritual, and religious beliefs and practices of the family. While revealing the information in light of these needs, the physician then checks for understanding and expresses empathy. This is to the reverse of an emotion-centered approach, which is distinguished by the doctor expressing the sadness of the message and demonstrating an excess of empathy and sympathy. This technique reveals the least amount of hope and hinders considerable information exchange [82].

Several protocols have been proposed and tested in the literature. Buckman has written extensively on this subject, including his outstanding book, (How to Break Bad News: A Guide for Health Care Professionals). His criteria for delivering bad news include delivering it in person, finding out how much the patient knows, sharing the information ("aligning"), assuring the message is understood, planning a contract, and following through [83].

Fine RL [84], initiated a protocol with five phases. Phase 1, preparation, involves foundation of adequate space, communicating time struggles, being critical to patient needs, being critical to cultural and religious values, and being specific about the goal. Phase 2, information acquisition, includes asking what the patient knows, how much the patient wants to know, and what the patient believes about his or her condition. Phase 3, information sharing, by reassessment the protocol and teaching. Phase 4, information reception, allows for evaluating the information reception, clarifying any misunderstanding, and handling disagreements respectfully, while Phase 5, response, involves recognizing and acknowledging the patient's response to the information and closing the interview [84].

Handling war prisoners' wounds and other enemy

Military healthcare practitioners can face ethical confrontation when their own soldiers and enemy soldiers are treated during the battle, with limited resources.

They are officially obliged to treat enemy soldiers equally under the Geneva Convention, but in the field, providers still have certain judgment. The basic ethical dilemma posed in this situation is "whether military physicians or other military healthcare professionals, would disobey an order for them to fulfill their professional ethical obligations." Several considerations may count.

All healthcare workers are supposed to do what is ethical and legal. The conflict may be is the definition of what this means precisely. Some have, accordingly, called for a "military ethical hotline" so that healthcare workers in suspicion may call to get immediate answers to difficult situations. There are criteria for this in other circumstances. Doctors may call a judge or magistrate, for example, when a crisis should be resolved immediately. As of this time, there is no known military medical ethics hotline military healthcare providers can call for authoritative advice.

The Geneva Convention holds that military healthcare providers must manage wounded prisoners of war in a way equal to their own. However, the translation of this law is not always clear.

However, by the end, that all healthcare providers, when facing difficult ethical dilemmas, should follow their own principles as a last resort, with a willingness to accept reverse consequences, with preserving the ability to look at oneself in a mirror [85,86].

Second opinion, the ethical aspect

Second opinion by definition is opinion provided by another or other spine surgeons, use to determine whether the course of treatment recommended by the first surgeon is valid or require partial or even complete diversion from the initial suggestion. By law the patient has the right to ask for second opinion, whenever he is not convinced of the line of treatment offered, moreover, he can ask his treating physician to guide him for finding another expert to help him in giving opinion.

Some surgeons are not happy for this policy, and some patients are not happy to ask for second opinion through the same surgeon or even they don't want him to know that they will ask for a second opinion.

Ethically the surgeon should ask for second opinion when he face a spinal pathology and he feels not capable of offering solution because he isn't experienced in this particular field, even at the time of surgery when he find difficult, he should ask for a colleagues' help without hesitation, so that no harm will touch the patient. If he don't ask for second opinion, and take a wrong decision, whenever pre-operative, intra-operative or even post-operative, when complications develops, he is guilty by sin of omission and commission.

Second opinion is a very practical, and required even by the most experienced surgeon, because no one knows everything. By second opinion you share free with the brain of your colleague, also this strengthen the colleague to colleague relationship and certainly improve the service offered to the patient which is the goal and the target of all spine surgeons. It's better to get the second opinion at the initial stage of disease, making use of the time factor, before it becomes too late to rectify the wrong decision or wrong treatment offered. Second opinion give a peace of mind to the surgeon and patient alike, and spare the surgeon from suing (visiting the court).

Ethically, the first surgeon should be informed without hesitation so that the decision of the treatment can be transferred (with all important documents) to the second surgeon. Always much better to keep the second opinion assign from wife, brother, friends, and other faraway, because they are really faraway from spine surgery. Two provisional opinions always better than one because two brains are much better than one brain.

One fact should be realized, that the clinical status, imaging, and investigations may change when consulting the second surgeon, this is probably one explanation for the difference between the first and second opinions.

Some surgeons in difficult spine pathology are asking routinely for a second opinion, even when they pretty sure at their management, on the assumption which is to keep the devil away and leave no room for the questioning and judging.

Common reasons to get a second opinion include suggestion for surgery as a treatment rather than conservative, without clear explanation why non- surgical treatment won't work?

Nassens in Mayo Clinic [87], confirmed that as many as 88 percent of those patient who came for second opinion, go home with a new refined diagnosis changing their care plan and potentially their lives. Conversely only 12 percent receive confirmation that the original diagnosis was complete and correct, also he confirmed that more than one out of every five referral patient may be completely (and) in correctly diagnosis.

Usually patients might want to see another doctor for confirming the diagnosis, to be sure of having the best treatment, and the doctor was not easy to ask about details. The advantage of seeing another doctor may include feeling reassured, that the second opinion was identical to the first, and having different choice to choose when the second doctor did not advise operation.

The second opinion is not always honey and milk, sometimes creates confusion, moreover, delays starting the treatment, additional cost, or getting difficulties in reaching the second doctor.

To sum up: The second opinion is ethically approved, and the patient is legally have the right to ask for. In sometime it is ethically required from the spine surgeon to guide the patient for second opinion, and also better always if he ask for second opinion in complex spine surgery or even in second spine surgery.

VI. Ethics of complications in spine surgery

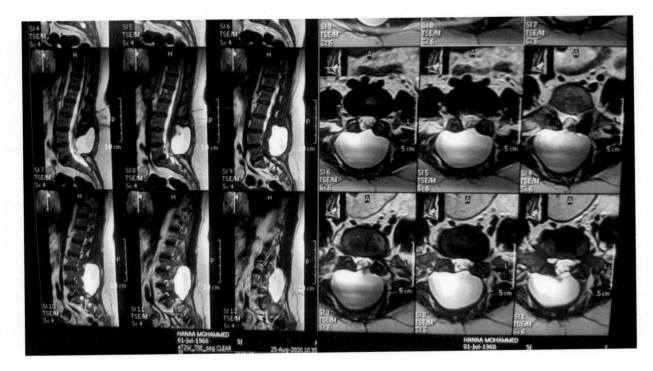

One of the complexities of spine surgery, is that the complications are inevitable. The frequency of complications is dependent on many reasons, like the nature of the underlining pathology, the experience of the surgeon, human error, technical failure, anatomical variations, unexpected biological responses, or any combination of these. In the majority of cases, there are negative consequences to the patient, of varying degrees or severity.

Complications are usually assessed and documented only by the medical staff directly involved in the treatment of the patient, and certain bias cannot completely excluded [88].

The input of the patient is seldom considered in connection with complications. This is an ethical point that should considered whenever complication appear, because the patient is the best judge to tell the reality of the surgical outcome. The variety of methodologies for assessing adverse events, may be one of the reasons for a wide-ranging complication rates reported in the literature for spine surgery, it's difficult to explain the variable incidence of 0-50% of complications for the same procedure in different papers [89]. Complications are by definition, something that should not occur and generally provoke a search for a reason or reasons behind.

The ethics start in the informed consent, where patients should be informed by every details, particularly, the expected complications, this should be done in a gentle way, and by conversation, understandable by the patient. The more the complications, the more the surgeon being to divulge them. Truth telling and openness, will certainly make the patient obedient, and cooperative, after the incidence of complications.

It's vital to differentiate between errors performed by the surgeon, i.e. induced by the surgeon, and complications, which is sometimes arises as a consequence of the pathological process.

Some surgeons, when they make a mistake, may attempt to disguise it by calling the error surgical complications, this behavior is not accepted ethically. This deceptive surgeon should specify that the complication was error, he is responsible about.

The junior surgeon has the right to improve his capabilities, this should be done under strict supervision, and to start with minor surgeries, and with time, the senior surgeon upgrades the junior.

The patient needs to be informed who will perform the surgery, and even the names of the assistant and other staff in the team.

If the treatment is beyond surgeons' capabilities, he is supposed to refer the patient to more experienced surgeon, who is capable of handling the patient probably. Some surgeons because of the aging process, physically being not capable to perform spine surgeries, here, he supposed to stop this career, and to leave the practice for the younger generation. For this surgeon, it's better to stop practicing the stressful surgeries, that produce a physical and mental exhaustion, and threatens the patients' life.

Spine surgeon should consider giving rest to the team in between the operations, to reduce boring and exhaustion. All theater equipment, better to be checked, or double checked, to be sure of its perfection prior to surgery. Good communications with the operating room staff, will make the work smooth and pleasing in the theater.

When complications occurs, the surgeon should have a moral obligation to minimize them as much as possible, and to avoid repeating them in future. If complications happen, the patient must be informed about the extent of the damage. And the progress in the near future, and if the surgeon has part of this event again, the patient informed about.

After the development of complications, there will be a definitive change in the patient psyche, which needs special care, sympathy and empathy from the treating physician. It's an ethical duty of the surgeon to transfer his complications' experience to his colleagues, by sharing in local, national, or even international conferences, or publish his experience in the medical journals. By doing so, a reduction in complications incidence may expect.

Complications may arise repeatedly from incompetent colleagues, in this case, there is moral obligation to advise him directly, provided that the patient was kept away from this colleagues' meeting. If the colleague repeating the same mistakes, or making serious situation, in that case a higher authority, such as professional body must be informed to find a solution.

Complications lead to delay in patients' discharge, so long occupation of the hospital beds, redo surgery may be required, and this will leads to economic burden.

Patients may entitled to a legal remedy and financial compensation in the event of negligent surgical complications.

It's preferable not to refer patients to centers or hospitals where the surgeon having a share in, and if so, it's better to inform the patient about this issue. This will increase the trust between the patient and his treating physician.

If the primary handling and care given for the patient prior to surgery were utmost and perfect, this will reduce anxiety, tension, and apprehension of the patient.

Finally, the ethical dilemma should not be ignored, and the relationship between the surgeon and patients should be maintained. Also, a financial support to the patient may be required, to reduce his burden after the development of complications. A share from the surgeons' side in this issue, will be very much appreciated [90].

VII. Medical negligence

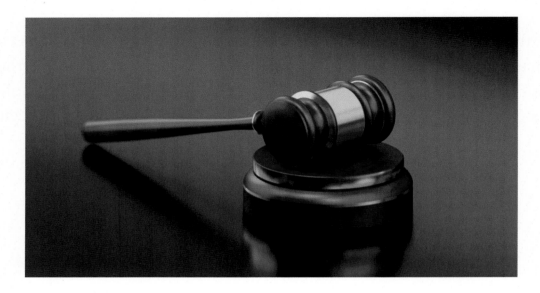

The medical profession is considered a noble profession because it helps in preserving human life. We believe life is God given. Thus, a doctor stands in the scheme of God as he supposes to carry out His command. A patient usually addresses a doctor/hospital based on his/ its reputation. Patient's expectations are of two-fold: doctors and hospitals are supposed to express medical treatment with all the knowledge and skills at their standards and secondly they will not do anything to harm the patient in any manner whether in a form of negligence, carelessness, or reckless attitude of their staff. Though a physician may not be able to save his patient's life at all times, he is proposed to utilize his specific knowledge and skills in the most appropriate manner keeping in mind the interest of the patient who has entrusted his life to him. Therefore, it is also anticipated that a practitioner would conduct necessary investigation or seeks a report from the patient. Moreover, except in emergency, he obtains informed consent of the patient prior to proceeding with any major treatment, surgical operation, or even invasive investigation. When the practitioner or the hospital struggle to perform this task, it is essentially a tortious obligation. A tort is a civil violation (right in rem) as against a contractual obligation (right in personam) an interference that might lead to judicial intervention by way of awarding damages. Therefore, a patient's right to receive medical care from physicians and hospitals is absolutely a civil right. This partnership will be formed as a contract to a large degree because of informed consent, fee charging, and performance of surgery/ providing treatment, etc. while retaining essential elements of tort [91].

There are two types of medical negligence; civil and criminal. In civil medical negligence, the physician earns a duty of care to the patient, and due to the breach of that care, the patient receives damage (physical or mental) where the damage was caused as a result of the breach of that duty. The standard of proof in civil medical negligence is (Balance of probability), that is more than 50% certainty.

When the negligent behavior is frank, ignorant, impetuous and not taking in consideration the life and safety of the patient, it is managed as criminal medical negligence and the standard of proof is (Beyond reasonable doubt) that is almost 100% certainty [92].

Applying ethical conduct to reduce negligence

Moral values in patient safety are not separated from basic medical obligations. Negligence, by definition, is lack of offering proper medical service to the patients, this include all aspects of service, with adding the required sympathy. It's really hateful, that patient's pay, sometime, a big price and prolong suffering, because of a negligent health care provider.

We admit that offering medical service to some patients, like those with dementia, Alzheimer, or terminally ill patients with disseminated malignancy, is not that easy, but this does not mean that they will be ignored, or negligence is permitted for them.

Adherence to the medical and ethical principles will certainly reduce, to great extent, falling in the trap of ignorance and negligence.

Negligence is based on the principle that a person must take a reasonable care to avoid act or omission, which would be likely to harm any person.

Negligence is confirmed when the risk was significant, leading to change in the patients' health, so a reasonable person would have to take precautions.

Negligence is a breach in the care and treatment offered. The possibility and risk of patient death occurring due to a preventable medical accident, while receiving health care, is estimated to be 1 in 300, to be compared with the avian accidents i.e. risk of dying while travelling by airplane, which is 1 in 3 million [93].

Negligence may start with the first meeting, when the patients' complain is not considered seriously, or even ignored. This may affect achieving the diagnosis. Then lacking the proper physical examination, which is consider a vital part in achieving diagnosis. Next to this, is ordering the specifically required investigations to achieve the definitive diagnosis. Overseeing, or even ignoring the results of investigations is a real negligence.

In emergency condition, a serious follow up of the results of investigations indicates seriousness and utmost care service, which is supposed to be comprehensive.

When writing the line of treatment, it's vital to consider seriously the emergency conditions that need urgent surgery, like spinal cord injuries, spinal cord compression, spinal infection that lead to epidural abscess, or a ruptured intervertebral disc with acute neurological deficit, or cauda equina syndrome, where the time factor is very vital. Wasting time in the above examples is non-ethical, and consider as ignorance in the eye of law.

The delay in treatment in general, has been associated with poor patients' outcome, and should be avoided at all cost. This is regarded as sub-standard of care. Asking for second opinion in complex spine pathology is considered as a real ethical conduct. As a spine surgeons, we have to maintain and ensure continuity of care, by providing communications between all health professionals, regarding patient health progress, and ethically, we have to follow the appearance of recent advances in patient care, to offer the best possible treatment, staying on the old regimen is rejected ethically.

Serious follow up of the patients' status is mandatory, it's un-ethical to leave the follow up to the junior staff, and what's worse than this, is to leave the follow up to the care of nursing staff.

Patients' records needs a very special care. Ignoring the records should be rejected. Records may be used to demonstrate accountability within the service, and if required in the court, records is considered as integral part of patient care. Records must include all details of the patients' condition.

The common documentation errors are;

➢ Wrong chart
➢ Wrong patient
➢ Inaccurate record
➢ Incomplete record
➢ Poor grammar and punctuation record
➢ Long unnecessary details
➢ Not adding the results of investigations and imaging to the record.

Good documentation can save health care providers from so many troubles, which include going to the court. Documentation protects the doctor, and the patient, alike. Messy, illegal documentation can cause misinterpretation. The consequence may be prosecution for negligence or a break of duty care.

The ethics committee jobs are to;

➢ Enhance learning solutions for the sophisticated medical technology
➢ Prevent abuse of human subject
➢ Increase the ethical concerns for health care providers, and also in educating the publics.

> ➤ Protect the patient's rights, and promote the ethical dimension of the health cars decision.

Depending on the above mentioned duties of the ethical committee, it is very vital to have the committee in all medical centers, because it's a safety valve for the health care providers and the patients.

Patients' safety is considered as a genuine part in ethical principle, which is considered as care quality indicator [94].

Based on the Iranian health care professional code of ethical conduct, it's expected that all patients be treated with dignity, and be protected from any possible harm [95].

The realism of patients' safety requires the provision and implementation of a professional code of ethics in addition to the scientific back ground.

Activity partnership with patient's family may be high yield approach to detect and prevent medical errors [96].

When errors were caused by inappropriate pattern of providing hospital service, it's better to inform the patient about all details in honest and clear language, and also it's required to give the patient enough time to express his feeling and his anger, which is an expected natural response from the patient side. The response of the patient will be worse if the hospital hide the reality.

Honest apology is required from the healthcare providers, and the victim of negligence is supposed to be fairly compensated. No point to disclose errors which did not affect the patients' health.

Protection of the staff will encourage them to report the incidents. But the patients' right must be protected under any condition, and it's above all.

Ethical aspects of unnecessary surgery

A well-known fact is that millions of patients all over the globe, every year fall under the knife without any reason, with millions of dollars spent unnecessarily. Some end up with painful complications, and some even die.

Unnecessary surgery by definition, is any surgical intervention that is either not needed, not indicated, or not in the patients' best benefit, when weigh against other available options [97].

In 1976, the American Medical Association (AMA) claiming that there were "2.4 million unnecessary operations performed on Americans at a cost of $3.9 billion and that 11,900 patients had died from unneeded operations [98].

The Harvard University School of Public Health, established that as many as 1.3 million Americans suffer disabling injury in the hospital yearly, and 198,000 of those may result in death. About 10 % of spinal fusion procedures paid for by Medicare in 2011 were unnecessary, with a cost of 157 million dollars [99,100].

The rate of medical harm occurring in the US is established to be over 40,000 harmful and/or lethal error every year [101].

A Cincinnati doctor did needless spinal surgeries to improve bone graft device [102].

The estimated figure for the unnecessary surgical operations all over the world varies from 30%-70%, performed for profit or corporate target of these hospitals [103].

Nancy Epstein and Donald Hood in 2011[104], found that during a one-year period, 47 [17.2%] of 274 spinal consultations seen by a single neurosurgeon were scheduled for "unnecessary surgery", although their neurological and radiographic findings were not abnormal.

So, obviously the story of unnecessary surgery is not rare, and the bad impact of it reflects on the patients and the economy.

They also discovered that out of the 45 patients, 13 of them were suffering from severe psychiatric disorders, 10 patients with morbid obesity, 10 with elevated cholesterol, 8 have diabetes, 7 have

Table 1: Major co-morbid factors in 29 [62%] of 47 patients scheduled for unnecessary spinal surgery [104].

Comorbidities	Patients No.
Hypertension	16
Severe psychiatric disorder [Bipolar]	13 [2]
Morbid obesity	10
Elevated cholesterol	10
Diabetes	8
Asthma	7
Smoker	3
Thyroid disease	3
Ulcers	3
Cardiac stents	3
Sleep apnea	2
Benign prostatic hypertrophy	2
Breast CA	2
Prostate CA	2
Peripheral vascular disease	2
Lupus	1
Sarcoidosis	1
Multiple sclerosis	1
Fibromyalgia	1
Chronic obstructive pulmonary disease	1
Peripheral europathy	1

asthma, 3 were heavy smokers, and a lot of chronic diseases like malignancy, multiple sclerosis... etc. table [1]. This obviously indicates that the primary clinical evaluation is insufficient, and below standards [104].

Depending on the above details, there is a real increase in the number of unnecessary surgery all over the world.

This number should be reduced to the minimum possible for the interest of our dear patients, as well as for the interest of reducing medical costs. Also more understanding of the need for spinal surgery is required.

There are many reasons behind the unnecessary surgeries, like, on the top of the list, is the financial incentive (greed), followed by lack of experience, ignorance, and stupidity, the pressure of the manufacturers of the drugs, instruments, fixation materials and other implants, are all playing probably a major role in the unethical conducts.

To avoid or minimize such interventions, special emphasis is required to implant the ethical aspect in all curriculum of both undergraduate and postgraduate students, and even after that, in all medical life. Ethics should be a fixed part of the continuous medical education all over the globe.

Strict and rigid law, with punishment for the non-ethical conduct, will definitely stop this malpractice, or decrease it to minimum.

Unnecessary surgery or even over surgery may be related to money oriented society, which will press hard on spine surgeons to gain their side towards their products, or toward their private hospitals. This obviously will increase all forms of malpractice.

Re-evaluation of the standard indications for spine surgeries, may help to reduce the incidence of unnecessary surgery. Also, emphasizing the policy of second opinion, or revision of any decision for surgery by the ethics committee, will certainly put a limit for any unacceptable malpractice.

Patients' education to ask for second opinion, whenever surgery is suggested as a solution, and to ask for details of the operation, and what is the alternatives, is also required.

We have to admit that the majority of spine surgeons work hard to diagnose and manage patients in a responsible, professional, and ethical manner consistent with the evidence available. Taking into serious consideration, the social and psychological background, the medico-legal context, and the ambiguous clinical examination, sadly, there are still, though they are few, spine surgeons, never stop practicing the unnecessary surgery, like over diagnosis, extensive surgery, unnecessary expensive, and potentially dangerous, leading to morbidity, mortality, or loosing huge money.

To sum up: To stop unnecessary surgery, which is unethical conduct, we need to:

Halt the companies from interference with clinical approach.

Educate spine surgeons by continuous medical education (CME), how to adhere to the ethical aspect of spine surgery.

Educate the patients to ask for second opinion, and to ask the decision makers about alternatives.

VIII. Commercialization of spine practice

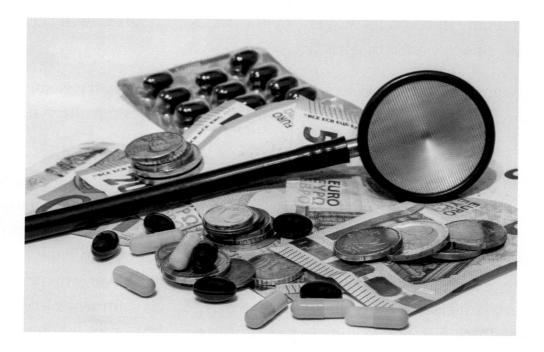

Commercialization is simply; to apply methods of business for profit. It is changing the scientific practice in to business. Or it's the organization of something in a way intended to make a profit. Also it's the process of introducing new products in the market, whenever the new products is developed by a company.

In spinal surgical practice, the commercialization is quite evident. The producers companies of the spinal instruments is increasing, day by day, with a strong competition to master the spinal practice. Every day there is a new modification, which needs a new set of instruments to implant the fixator, or cage, with a new rise in the price.

Despite the extensive trials of the companies to buy the brain of spine surgeons, and drive the results of their approach or operative procedures to their benefit, by offering big incentive and discount to them. Spine surgeons should always remember that they have the responsibility to provide the utmost care to their patients, without the pressure or the effect of the manufacturing companies. Strict supervision of the ministry of health is required to keep the companies influence far away from spinal practice, which should remain clean and honest.

Leading companies in spine practice, and others are spending millions of dollars for marketing of their products. A report on Forbs, claimed that Medtronic spends more money on selling and promotions, and less on building [105].

No doubt, the companies played a major rule in the progress of spine surgery, they contributed in the development of the computer assisted surgery, robotic surgery, surgical microscope, spinal fixation systems, and other implants, which are beyond count. Another fact, which we cannot deny, is their contribution in education, fellowships, supervising spine conferences, running courses, and so many activities, probably, without them no advancement can be achieved. This contributions has been used as a venue for marketing their products, and making a sound name in the field of spine surgery.

All researchers supervised by companies end up with positive results to their end. Exchange of benefit is the green flag always raised by the companies. They keep making a new revision, though minor, to produce a new set of instruments, which is totally different from sets of other companies. So there is no similarity, in that case, only their specific products can be used, simply we can call this company selfishness. The other end of the story, is that medical device companies focused on simplifying the surgical act by designing, developing, and promoting safe and effective solutions to spine surgery, and operating room technology, hopefully they combined low cost and efficiency in their products.

The last decade has brought a new challenges to the traditional practice, which is related, to some extent, to what we call a commercial spine surgeon, those whose target is to support companies on the behalf of the patients, this is ethically rejected and never acceptable.

We have to be aware not sliding from medical service to commercial service. And also we have to be aware of procedure-driven marketing.

Corporates are always send their non-physician executive to introduce their products as a gold standard, and they try their best to invariably divert the decision to their benefit.

The basic promises for separation is the divided loyalty, and impaired confidence between the interest of corporation and the needs of the patients [106].

The companies always announce amazing and very attractive sentences about their products in their websites, by doing so, they convince patients and divert their attention to certain implant, fixation system, or procedure. This will create difficulty for the spine surgeon to perform what is in his mind, which might be contradictory to the corporate suggestions. The common denominator appears to be on emphasis on company profit, over quality and patient safety.

Patients are seeking medical advice, not a proprietary commercial product that any licensed physician can prescribe. Sadly, copywriting medical contributions have even founds its way into academic medicine.

Critical analysis and evaluation of the new product is mandatory. This includes the scientific bases, the obvious therapeutic difference, and any marketing advantages [107].

It is always better to wait the test of time, which does indicate the goodness of the new products.

Sometimes the companies emphasize on names, that's making use of notable names in spine practice to facilitate marketing, sadly, by sharing them a percentage of the profits, gifts, discounts, and other ways to convince them supporting the company products. State health care statutes prohibit doctors from marketing unsubstantiated claims of superiority [108,109].

Maximize profit and sidestep, such issue as credentialing and safety guidelines are mandating by our professional societies, the common denominator appears to be emphasis on profit over quality and safety [110].

Conflicts of interest

In spine surgery practice, the relationship between spine surgeon in practice, and drug and medical devices companies, are extensive, this is because of the development of instruments, machines, fixators, and implants. This relation on many occasions serves the companies, rather than the patients. The companies spend millions of dollars as commissions and incentives for the spine surgeons, to support their products, even if it's not perfect. This is a real bias to the benefit of the companies rather than to the patients.

Certainly this is unethical attitude, and better to be resisted, to preserve the honesty.

The idea behind the conflict of interest is to restrict this ties to the companies, so the surgeons are obliged to mention in a clear language this relation with the companies, or any other source of financial support, and by doing so, he clarify the solidity of his clinical work, or clinical research.

The conflict of interest is mandatory in spine practice, because it may help to break the ties with the companies.

The spine surgeons and the responsibility to their patients

Patients' safety and benefit take precedence over any business concern. Our credibility with our patients should not be under estimated [106].

Our patients looks to us for truth and honesty, so we should not take these points lightly. Service is not interchangeable, patients are dissimilar, surgeons are unique in their capabilities, and techniques are individualized, so, what remains and what is on the top of everything is patients' benefit and safety with the minimum cost possible.

To sum up: the companies and corporate will come and go, what is good today is not necessarily will be also good tomorrow. We should not accept what's less than ideal from all directions. And never accept offers from companies to facilitate marketing of their products. Most researches that brings new drugs from bench to bedside are financed by pharmaceutical companies.

IX. Collegial Ethics

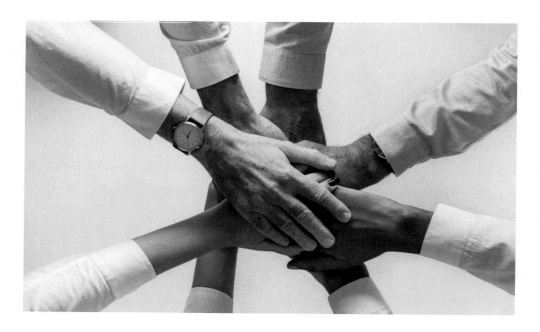

Ethics alive when you are ethical concern.

It is vital and essential for good and safe patient care that we have to work in harmony, respect, and mutual help with our dear colleagues in the same department, and with other health discipline. Whenever we work as a team, the relation should be similar to the football team. The ideal relations needs transparency, by which we enlarge, exchange of opinions, which is another vital point, justice in all aspect of the work, will spare us a lot of troubles.

Colleagues are friends in work time, but not necessary the best friends, friendship is required in work environment to preserve the patients' rights.

We have to show respect, not for them only, but also for their work ethics and ideas. If we are not happy about their ideas or work performance, we have to be gentle in handling this point.

It is also very important to avoid, totally, a gossip or the talk behind colleagues' back, if there is a problem with a colleague, it's preferable to handle it naturally, and confront him directly, everyone is equal, and should be treated as such. It's unethical to talk dawn with colleagues or disrespect them, on the contrary, we have to communicate with them in an open way, seriously willing to share ideas.

We have to learn how to compromise, because it's instrumented to success in work place. It's mandatory to listen carefully to colleagues, in order to produce positive work relations, and to open ears for their suggestions. Never let your colleagues feel that you are superior to them. Some social life activity sharing brings them closer together.

Trust between colleagues is required, because the trust is the foundation of the very good relationship.

Diversity in the work place is welcomed, but putting a blame on your colleagues' shoulder better to be avoided. It's better to stay always on the positive side, even with the junior doctors or the nursing staff. Setting a boundaries with the junior doctors or the nursing staff is required, in addition to the mutual respect. It's nice to be friendly and kind to them, we are professional and that work comes first.

Solving the problems which arises during work, better to be in the department, far away from the administration office.

Sadly, some colleagues don't understand the importance of working in harmony, the outcome of this is always bad, and reflected badly on offering utmost service to the patients. We have to convince such colleagues in a gentle way to make them feel the importance of team work, by offering constructive criticism, never talk down or disrespect them, offer guidance and positive reinforcement, showing them that we are advocate and willing to help to upgrade the patients' service.

We have to tackle discrimination when it arise, and encourage colleagues to do the same. In the same time we should challenge the behavior of colleagues who do not meet the required standards.

Exchange of patient referral will certainly strengthen the collegial relationship. So it's better to refer patients that lies outside your field of expertise, to colleagues with special interest in that particular field.

When we mentor junior colleagues, we have to keep positive, and remain loyal to them.

Unfortunately, the patients may disrupt the colleagues' relationship, by transferring incorrect message, sadly, some patients are really dishonest, and they behave like this intentionally. So it's better not to listen to them, and discuss the issue directly with the concerned colleague. Better not to lose a friend you see him every morning, because of a trouble maker patient, probably you will never meet him again.

We have to treat all colleagues fairly foster equality of opportunity, never allow the personal relationship with colleagues to be prejudiced by their own personal view about their lifestyle, gender, age, race, sexual orientation, belief or culture. It's unethical to discriminate against colleagues on any of those ground.

Always it's better not to make unfair remarks about the previous management in front of the patient. All communications between colleagues about the patients' condition should be on professional bases, purposeful, respectful, and consistent with the patients' benefit, and better to keep the patient away from the professional correspondence.

Many of our actions and reactions with our colleagues are instinctive. Using actions, compassion, fairness, and courage, in the pursuit of supportive position with colleagues is worth stressing [111].

Some colleagues may face problems, accusation, or difficult circumstances, so we have to help them, as we would to be helped. We need to develop a style and language of mutual support with each other.

In the eye of law, colleague is not guilty, until proven guilty. There is a difference between legal guilt and ethical guilt, even if the legal guilt was not confirmed, an ethical may be incurred [111].

Supporting colleagues must not mean we may perceive dander to ourselves, in this case, we better to stay out of it. This is true when a crime has been committed by a colleague, when support may not be appropriate. No support is offered to colleagues if this is against the patient's right, or it's harmful to the patient in any form.

Supporting colleagues in trouble time is required to avoid destructive acts. Timely help and effective collegial support would have made a difference, at least, in some cases, though the goal of collegial ethics is to actively support colleagues and to develop the skills needed to do so. Excessive fairness is required before trying to help colleagues, we have to study the case from all points of view [112].

Despite this and that, we should be pleasant and gorgeous to actively support colleagues, when they are in a trouble. This will enhance the quality of our work and our life.

When things are going smooth, and there are no conflicts or problems, it can be easy to support each other, but when there is a problem, which may be a personal failure, external attack, or a complex turn in one's professional career, we have to study the details of the case before sharing in the solution, because the trouble can be serious such as accusation or misconduct or black listing [112].

When serious accusation are made damage to the accused can persist in some form, even if the accused is vindicated [113].

Finally, what we have to do to our colleagues, is what we want them to do for us, in a similar situation.

Collogues relationship

Communicating effectively and building respectful relationships among one's medical colleagues is an important obligation in achieving the goals of Medicine and building trust and confidence in the profession.

Supporting colleagues in gaining competence and resolving disputes among colleagues is a vital feature of collegiality. Collegiality is the forgotten pillar of professionalism. It is time for all doctors to resurrect it for the benefit of patients, society and the profession.

Healthy collegiality

Healthy collegiality between physicians relies on reciprocal respect and trust with collaboration and cooperation of shared decision making for the benefit of the patients. The patients' maximum benefit and the aims of medicine, medical education and scientific research serve as the common purpose. The establishment of these principles should not only be developed but also assessed throughout the way of professional carrier.

Throughout any environments, even in emotionally stressful and difficult ones, doctors have to preserve the standard of respect for colleagues and certify that the trust and confidence in the profession is not battered by behavior or words. The features of the profession, integrity and honour, should be preserved always.

To preserve and encourage healthy collegiality, doctors not only need to know of collegial values and rules adminstrating the relationship, but should also be taught and encouraged to pracice healthy collegial professional behaviours [114,115].

Professional behaviors marking healthy collegiality:

➢ Maintains serenity during difficult communications with colleagues

➤ Supports and benefit exchange with colleagues when its possible

➤ Fulfilment allocated part of team duties

➤ Holds on additional work to assisst colleagues when needed and convenient

➤ Shares information and expertise with colleagues

➤ Produces a significant influence during conferences and clinical practice

➤ Confession in mistakes and admits personal responsibility for them

➤ Recognizes the assistances of others

➤ Encourages for colleagues

➤ Appreciative and responsive to power divergence in inter-professional communications

➤ Reacts accordingly to colleagues in trouble or impaired partners

➤ Recognize and express appropriate limits for inter-professional communications

➤ Upholds creative attitude and incentive during unexpected work consequences [114,115].

Unhealthy collegiality

Unhealthy collegiality is distinguished by stimulating similarity and preventing diversity, avoids dissent, discussion and constructive criticism by identifying them as disloyalty, and creates gratification of standards by ignoring malpractice and impaired colleagues. These performances will necessarily limit academic liberty and development, and leads to a culture of groupthink.

Groupthink occurs when a group desires organization and concurrence instead of the original common purpose:

➢ Shows difference as disloyalty
➢ Seeks negotiation and not consensus
➢ Makes pragmatic rather than practical decisions
➢ Disregard valid alternatives
➢ Rationalizes away risks [114-116].

Delegation, referral and handover

Delegation implicates that a health care professional asking another colleague to provide care on his behalf while he retain overall responsibility for the patient's care. Referral involves that a health care professional sending a patient to obtain opinion or treatment from another doctor or colleague. Referral commonly reflects the transfer (in part) of responsibility for the patient's care, usually for a specific time and for a particular purpose, such as care which is beyond your area of expertise. Handover is the procedure of transferring all responsibility to another health care professional. Important steps here involves [117]:

➢ Taking intelligent measures to ensure that the colleague to whom you delegate, refer or handover has the qualifications, experience, knowledge and skills to provide a qualified healthcare.
➢ Recognizing that when the healthcare professional delegate, although he will not be responsible for the decisions and actions of those to whom he delegate, he still responsible for the overall management of the patient, and for his decision to delegate.
➢ Always discussing adequate information about the patient and the treatment they need to ensure the persistent care of the patient.

Teamwork

Most physicians work tightly with a wide range of health care professionals. Patients' care is enhanced when mutual respect and efficient communication exist, and when healthcare providers understand each other's responsibilities, abilities, limitations and ethical codes. Teamwork should not alter a doctor's personal responsibility for professional conduct and the care provided. When working in a team, for improving the medical practice you may need:

➢ Recognizing your specific position in the team and accomplishing to the duties related to that role.

➢ Encouraging for a clear description of duties and responsibilities, including that there is a recognized team leader or coordinator.

➢ Communicating efficiently with other team members.

➢ Inform patients regarding to the duties of team members.

➢ Acting as a positive role model for team members.

➢ Recognizing the character and consequences of bullying and harassment, and working to eliminate such behavior in the workplace.

Coordinating care with other doctors

A qualified patient care requires coordination between all treating physicians. Good medical practice involves:

➢ Sharing all the relevant information in a timely manner.

➢ Enhancing the central coordinating position of the general practitioner.

➤ Supporting the importance of a general practitioner to a patient who does not already have one.

➤ Confirming that it is obvious to the patient, the family and colleagues who has crucial concern for coordinating the care of the patient.

X. The ethics of funding innovation, research, and other activities

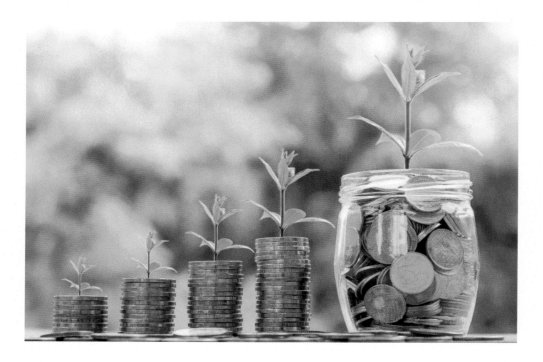

The performance of a research, or an innovative procedure is very expensive. This is one of the limitations in spine surgery. So, to improve research and innovation, there is a real need to find a funding source, provided that the funding source will not apply a pressure on the researchers or innovators to make the outcome to their interest, or serving their benefit. Nowadays we are all really facing this issue, which we have to stand against. So this condition should be fixed in advance. The source of funding with special emphasis on the neutrality of the work.

Finding the source of funding is not that easy, and may require invasive, and longtime search.

Funding for a research, innovative procedure or treatment, can be obtained from a variety of sources, like [118]:

Patient self-payment

Insurance companies usually will not cover the unproven treatments. Also it's not fair that the patient covers the cost of treatment when there is no scientific evidence for its application.

We may think of selecting patients based on their ability to pay, leading to a bias in which only wealthy patients are offered novel treatments. This is not justice, and patients would be selected for novel procedures solely based on their clinical status.

According to the code of medical ethics; "A physician shall support access to medical care for all people". So, ethically speaking, this source of funding is not recommended, and no patient will cover payment for an innovative procedure [118].

Insurance covering

Insurance companies usually do not support innovation and research, so the burden will be on the patient money sources. Usually the insurance company covers an FDA approved medicine, and not happy to cover a cost for the newly produced medicine [119].

Industry Funding

Obviously, researches and medical innovation, including in spine surgery, would not be possible today without the financial support of pharmaceutical companies and medical device manufacturers, so there is a real need for a partnership with industry to achieve a progress in the field of spine surgery.

It was proven that industry-funded research is more likely to report positive results, than non-industry funded work [120].

Collaboration between clinicians and industry researchers is unavoidable, but this collaboration is not without drawback, because some spine surgeons may have financial interest in the success of that technologies, with resultant bias, to the benefit of the company funding the research. This bias is the result of improper conduction or interpretation of the research. So, it's better to avoid this support, or reduce the sharing to the least possible [121].

Philanthropy

This comes from individual donations, patient support groups, charitable foundations, or other sources. It is at the opposite end of the spectrum from financially motivated industry-driven funding.

Many advantages behind this type of support, it is freeing the innovators from many potential conflicts of interest, easier to achieve, and usually given with no restrictions or limitations on how it can be spent, other than the reasonable assumption that it is put to good use. They do not usually personally stand to profit, other than perhaps fulfilling a personal desire to help cure a disease or make the world a better place. But it should be also used for the benefit of the patients' health. So probably, this type of financial support is the preferable one [122].

Academic/Institutional Support

Universities support the research for education, and may be for other reasons (like a desire on the part of the institution to profit off of patents, boost their reputation, and attract desirable researchers and physicians). But usually not very much this small donation may stimulate other institutes to support research funding.

Hospitals also contribute to funding research financially, if the research will be a source of money in the future.

This source of donation is acceptable, provided that there is no personal benefit [123].

Government Grants

In the United States, the second-largest source of funding for medical research and development is the government [124].

Governmental funding is very vital, and usually directed to the patients' benefit solely, so there will be no bias in the final outcome. In other words, there is not much concern that financial concerns will influence the outcomes of research. It is true that political pressures could affect the distribution of money to particular research topics; however, the degree to which this occurs is likely less than the forces at work in the private sector. There are also professional pressures on innovators who win grants to "publish or perish," to produce short term outcomes, and to win more and more grants as their careers progress. But still this is a good source of support [125].

Other sources

Humanitarian society may help in funding. The crowd funding medical expenses incurred during innovation should be avoided if possible [126].

Charitable trust may also support research. So it is vital to be sure from where the money comes.

The innovator should be proactive in avoiding conflict of interest.

Irrespective of money source, innovation will inherently come with some degree of pressure for certain results. While innovators should avoid conflicts, funding sources should also be cognizant of and resist the temptation to create conflicts, whether they are financial, professional, or some other types of pressure to get certain results from the researchers. All funding sources should have the mission of improving patient care, and they should not spoil this mission by looking for personal gain.

XI. Ethics Committee

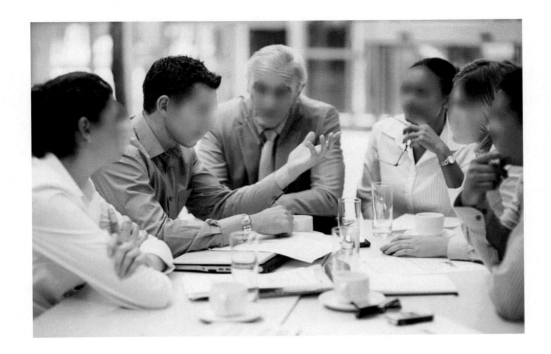

It is a committee of board of reliable pioneers, experienced personnel with special interest in the ethical aspects of spine surgery. Basically to promote the ethical aspects of spine surgery, and responsible for the code of ethics and conduct, and other ethical guidance within the society.

The committee cornerstone works, are protecting the rights, safety, dignity, and well-being of the people participating in the research, and protecting the researcher himself.

Moreover the committee promotes ethical practice, provide guidance on ethical matters related to spine surgery. Also perform regular symposiums and courses at regular intervals, supervise all researches in the vicinity. No research will be performed without getting a written permission from the committee. The committee other important task is publishing educational booklets about the ethical rules of research to the researchers, and even to the public, and providing ethical case consultations, rectify ethical works, supervise and follow research performance, deliver training and support to the researchers.

The committee usually follow a standard guidance to avoid fraud, plagiarism, and fabrication.

The committee supposed to offer the efficient and robust ethics review service, that maximize health services and health research, and maximize patients' benefit, and in the same time preventing harm, and offering benefit and safety to the respondents and researchers.

All research protocols must be submitted for review to the committee, which consists at least of five members of experienced spine surgeons, with good ethical background, and they are fully aware of the drawbacks and negative points in spine practice. So that, they keep the patients away from harm, as a result of treatment or research project. They have the right to reject a research or treatment, which is not in accordance with the ethical criteria. Also they have the authority to follow the progress of the research or treatment, to confirm continuity or stop the process if it was improperly done, or not following the standard rules agreed upon with the committee.

Researchers are supposed to write to the ethical committee a report about the progress of the research, any drawbacks, end of the study, study termination, and study extension, if required. The committee should seriously analyze the report raised, and put down their remarks.

They are supposed to provide annual report, with details about their positive impact, with remarks about how to improve the performance of the committee. Preferable to change the members of the committee every three years.

We think it's very vital to establish this committee in every institute, hospitals, and universities, to rectify and improve the function, and in the same time establishing the principles of ethics which is very vital to every aspect of daily work [127-132].

Ethics in research and innovation

Research and innovations plays a major role in the advancement of any science. This is particularly true in spine surgery, due to the rapid development, and the big participation of commercial companies, trying always to buy the brains of spine surgeons, by offering big incentive, also the tremendous advances in technology that have tremendously expanded what can be done and what cannot be done. So ethics is very vital to protect spine surgery from misconduct and fallacies, which is usually serving, or acting on the benefit of companies of implants and instruments. Moreover is the pressure of the pharmaceutical industries.

All research projects and innovations must be admitted to the local ethical committee, with every tinny details about the project. A permission from the ethical committee is mandatory before starting the research. The duty of the ethical committee is to critically analyze the project, before giving the accurate decision [133].

Also, it's their job to follow the progress the project, and to say yes to continue, or no to terminate the work, if it's not ethically approved.

Research ethics provide guidelines for the responsible conduct of research, in addition it educates and monitors scientists conducting research to ensure high ethical standards. The ethical rules are required in all aspect of the research, like project preparation, design, methods, analysis of the results, and telling the truth as it is. No fraud or fabrication. So, a standard ethical frameworks serves patients and community.

Various ethical cods mentioned the vital principles of research ethics. We consider the following points which was mentioned by Adil E. Shamoo and David B. Resnik, very vital to have ethically approved research [133-135].

Honesty

Is very much required to end up with a fruitful outcome. Honesty involves all aspect of the research. Researchers should never fabricate, falsify, or misrepresent the data, never deceive colleagues, research sponsors, or public.

Integrity

Keep your promises and agreements act with sincerity, research should be comprehensive and integral

Objectivity

Always better to avoid bias in experimental design, data analysis, data interpretation, publication, peer review, personnel decisions, grant writing, expert testimony, and other aspects of research where objectivity is expected or required. Disclosure should be included.

Carefulness

Errors and negligence are not acceptable. Carefully and critically the work must be examined. Keep good records of research activities, such as data collection, research design, consent forms, and correspondence with agencies or journals.

Openness

Sharing data, results, ideas, tools, materials, and resources with colleagues to accept criticism and new ideas.

Intellectual property

All patents, copyrights, and other forms of intellectual property, need to be equally distributed for all contributors to the research.

Confidentiality

Always better to protect confidential communications, such as papers or grants submitted for publication, personnel records, proprietary information, and records that identify individual research subjects or patients.

Publications

Publish to advance research and science, and distribute the knowledge, it is hateful to be selfish.

Responsible mentoring

Help is required to mentor and advice students, promote their welfare and help them to make decision.

Respect to contributors

Mutual respect is required between colleagues in the research group, to make the research smooth and quite.

Social responsibility

Research should never include any form of harm or danger to the community.

Nondiscrimination

All sharing in the research should receive equal rights in all aspects, depending on their amount of contributions. No points of difference.

Competence

Competence is mandatory and required to be maintained throughout the process. This will improve the professional competence and experience through lifelong education and learning.

Legality

All laws and institutional regulations must be respected. No rule breaking under any condition.

The harm to human and animal sharing in the research project must be minimized to the least possible. Respect for human dignity, privacy, and autonomy should be preserved.

Emanuel et al, described seven requirements for ethical research to be in the best shape possible, these include social or scientific value, scientific validity for subject selection, favorable risk-benefit ratio, independent review, informed consent, and respect for potential and enrolled subjects which are more or less similar to the requirements suggested by David Resnik [133-135]. Some activities are considered un-ethical by most researchers like:

➤ Publishing the same paper in many journals.
➤ Submitting the same paper in many journals.
➤ Applying for prize or patent without informing the shared researchers.
➤ Adding name as contributor without real contribution.
➤ Using inappropriate statistical technique in order to enhance the significance of the research.
➤ Stretching the truth for job application or curriculum vita.
➤ Changing or modifying the result for a personal intention or benefit.
➤ Conducting a review of literature that fails to acknowledge the contributors or other people in the field, or relevant prior work.
➤ Making significant deviations from the research protocol, approved by the ethical committee.
➤ Not reporting the adverse events.
➤ Stealing books, supplies, or data.
➤ Deliberately overestimating the clinical significance of a new drug, in order to obtain economic benefit.

The above mentioned twelve points are considered unethical by several researchers, some might be even considered illegal. Most of those would also violate different professional ethics codes, or institutional policies.

A special ethical consideration is required for a number of controversial topics, like human embryonic stem cell research, cloning, genetic engineering, and research involving human or animal subjects.

So, the spine surgeons must be more serious than before, to ensure that they are maintaining the highest standard possible in research. Methodology, human dignity, patient beneficence, non-maleficence, and justice, are fundamental values that should not be forgotten for every clinical research.

Finally, no research can be considered comprehensive if it's not obey the ethical or institutional requirements.

XII. The Learning Curve in Spine Surgery

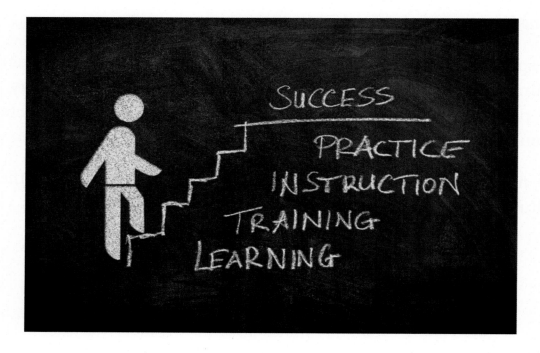

Spine surgery is considered as one of the most difficult surgeries, due to the anatomical complexity of the spine, variety of pathologies with high risk of recurrence, high risk of complications, and frequent association with comorbidities, specially, in elderly patients, in addition to the difficult surgical technique. So, it's not that easy to master spine surgery in a short period of time. Probably, several years is required. New technologies are evolving every frequently because of the commercialization of spine surgery. So, a learning curve is required for both, the senior and the junior surgeons.

The learning curve by definition: is the improvement of learning of a new procedure, or performance of a new technique, which tends to improve with the experience and time, in addition to the personal capabilities, which is probably unique, and differs from person to person. Some persons were born to be a surgeons, while others are not.

It's vital for the junior to know his capabilities, in order to continue the journey of spine surgery, and also it's the job of the senior supervisor to inform the junior if he is fit to continue, or to change to other medical or surgical specialty.

Improvement is expected with increasing experience, this concepts applies a cross the full spectrum of medical specialties and surgical procedures. If no improvement happen, this either indicates lack of capabilities, or lack of the serious interest. There should be no learning curve as far as patients' safety is concerned. Patients are not experimental animals for learning, under any conditions. In that case, patients should not be exposed to surgeons operating during early phase of their learning curve [136].

Sadly, still some patients suffering from morbidity, or even become crippled, because the surgery was performed by an unexperienced surgeon. This story is probably occurring every day, and all over the globe.

Probably the curve below (figure 1) is a useful guide for the perfection of performance is a modification of the curve suggested by Hooper.

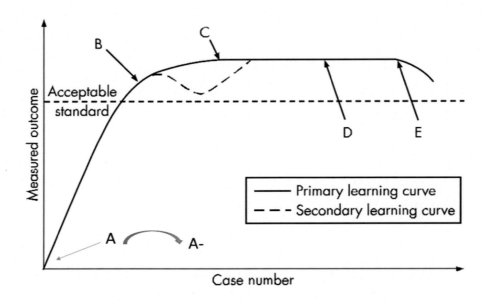

Figure 1; surgical learning curve.

A   Slow start
A- The unfit junior, could not be manage to continue
B   Gradual improvement with time
C   Peak rise
D   Plateau status
E   Falling down again, because of aging process

Dotted line for temporary decline, due to overconfidence, or new procedures (new development).

Years of experience of clinical practice and doing surgeries are required for the surgeon to pass from the low level to a higher level (upgrading) experience [137].

Learning curve graphically represent the relationship between learning effort and the result of surgery. The speed and efficacy increased by time, and it's not that easy to assess the clinical performance, the assessment measures includes; proper dissection respecting normal tissue, dissection layer by layer on anatomical bases. Operative time, blood loss, proper hemostasis. While in the post-operative period, assessment depends on patient's outcome, like analgesia requirement, transfusion requirement, absence of pre-operative symptoms and signs, duration of hospital stay, morbidity, mortality, and patient satisfaction.

Though surgical procedures differs depending on the pathology, dissection on a virgin tissue differs very much from dissection on a non-virgin tissue. Also the presence of congenital anomalies and comorbidities should be considered. The manual dexterity varies between surgeons. The old standard surgeons prefer to continue to feel that comfort lies in the old procedures, some of them not even looking for change, because learning a new procedure even for an established consultant requires an effort to improve the learning curve. We have to learn from every case and evolve our technique.

Surgeons have always recognized the concept of learning curve when undertaking a new procedure. Suboptimal results due to lack of experience for the new development, is never accepted.

How to improve the learning curve?

Introducing a new procedure should be in a structured way, that incorporate formal training course, cadaveric dissection, visiting experienced surgeon, watching live operation by the expert surgeons, and assisting actively in that surgery. Specialized training in the form of observationship, fellowship, simple or advanced simulation training, and watching operative videos.

It's always better to have a senior surgeon standing opposite side to guide the junior and take over when he feels that the junior is not capable of performing the procedure effectively. The policy of see one and do one is not applicable in spine surgery.

Also, to improve the learning curve, we need a good theoretical background, and patience, because the time factor is very vital to improve the curve. We have to remember that (foolish who learn from his mistakes, he should learn from mistakes of the others).

The patients should be spared from the learning curve, so the learning curve should never be at the expense of patient's health. Our duty in providing health care is to get the risk and harm to the minimum, while, at the same time learning ourselves and teaching our colleagues and junior staff.

Spine surgeons are appointed after finishing the required time for training, and getting the specialized degree. Some of them are appointed with a shortness of the expert phase for a certain procedure [138].

Supervised training opportunities are very vital for the new consultants and juniors.

The newly appointed consultant must recognize the need for continuing the post accreditation training, structured appraisal, and senior mentors, are required to facilitate the good progress of the learning curve. So that acceptable outcome may be achieved and maintained. Assessment of the curve progress with appropriate feedback and testing from the senior surgeon is mandatory, though there is some diversity related to the outcome [137].

In regard to curve progress, it's vital to recognize that there is individual variation in the speed and learning uptake, some are outstanding, some are perfect, some are good, and some are below the required standard.

A decline in the curve progress is expected with advanced age, due to decrease in manual dexterity, eye sight, memory and cognition. This deterioration is outweighing the advantage of long experience, leading to a fall in the level of performance, so, restriction is required for the old seniors.

Temporary drop in the curve may happen due to overconfidence, or undertaking more difficult cases beyond surgeon's capabilities, resulting in laps in technique or judgment. So, the chairman should specify the surgery to the juniors or young consultants according to their level of experience, or location in the learning curve. It's better not to start with complicated and technically demanding procedures, like revision surgeries. Progression of the curve depends on how complex is the technique of the operation. Serial monitoring for the outcome of the specific procedure is required for the evaluation of the progress of the curve. It's better to appoint a senior spine surgeon to follow the curve progression of the juniors, by doing so, it's possible to estimate the location of the junior on the learning curve [139,140].

Suggests that to decide whether to adopt a specific new techniques, the following points should be considered:

➢ Does it improve the quality of care?
➢ The frequency of associated complications.
➢ Does the new technology improve the efficiency in delivering care? Does it save time, reduce time for medical or surgical errors, and have less staff required?
➢ Does the technology made a financial sense?

So before applying a new technology we have to evaluate its impact on patient's benefit.

Finally, we have to realize how much the quality of our patients' life will be better, rather than how much the junior doctors will be better, and how much we are capable of giving our patients a normal spine. The spine surgeon should ask himself, is he doing the best for his patients? Is he giving them the surgery that he would want to receive?

References

1   A. Steinberg. Encyclopedia of Jewish Medical Ethics (English Edition), Feldheim Publishers. Vol. II, 2003, pp. 389-404.

2   Sisir K. Majumdar. History of evolution of the concept of Medical ethics. Bulletin of the Indian Institute of History of Medicine (Hyderabad). 2003. 33(1):17-31.

3   Tatsuo Kuroyanagi. Historical transition in medical ethics— challenges of the world medical association. JMAJ 2013,56(4): 220–226.

4   Peter Singer. Ethics philosophy. Encyclpedia Britanica. https://www.britannica.com/topic/ethics-philosophy#ref59238. Accessed April 14, 2020.

5   T Halwani, M Takrouri. Medical laws and ethics of Babylon as read in Hammurabi's code (History). The Internet Journal of Law, Healthcare and Ethics. 2006 Volume 4 Number 2.

6   The Code of Hammurabi: The Best Rule to Manage Risk. Farnam Streat. https://fs.blog/2017/11/hammurabis-code. Accesses April 14, 2020.

7   Ralph Jackson. Doctors and diseases in the Roman Empire. 2016 Global-HELP Organization. PP 9-31.

8   Maimonides. https://en.wikipedia.org/wiki/Maimonides. Accessed April 14, 2020.

9   Fred Rosner. The physician's prayer attributed to Moses Maimonides. Bulletin of the History of Medicine. 41(5), 1967, pp. 440-454.

10   Joseph Jacobs, Isaac Broydé, Jacob Zallel Lauterbach. Moses Ben Maimon (Rambam; usually called Maimonides). http://www.jewishencyclopedia.com/articles/11124-moses-ben-maimon. Accessed April 14, 2020.

11   Ram Pande. Charaka-samhita. Shodhak. 2017, Vol.47:B, 140.

12   Ala Sh. Ali. Research misconduct and research ethics – II. Iraqi New Medical Journal January 2017;3(1).

13   Patuzzo Sara, Goracci Giada, Ciliberti Rosagemma. Thomas Percival. Discussing the foundation of Medical Ethics. Acta Biomed. 2018; 89(3): 343–348.

14   WMA Declaration of Geneva. https://www.wma.net/policies-post/wma-declaration-of-geneva/. Accessed April 14, 2020.

15   Wiesing U, Parsa-Parsi R. The World Medical Association Launches A Revision of the Declaration of Geneva. Bioethics. 2016 Mar;30(3):140.

16   Jonathan D. Moreno, Ulf Schmidt, Steve Joffe. The Nuremberg Code 70 years later. JAMA. 2017;318(9):795-796.

17   Nuremberg Code. http://broughttolife.sciencemuseum.org.uk/broughttolife/techniques/nurembergcode. Accessed April 9, 2020.

18   Bulletin of the World Health Organization, 2001, 79 (4).

19   Ramin Walter Parsa-Parsi. The revised declaration of Geneva, a modern-day physician's pledge. JAMA, 2017: 318(20).

20   Stephen G. Post. Compassionate Care. J IMA. 2011 Dec; 43(3): 148–159.

21   Christina M. Puchalski, Stephen G. Post, Richard P. Sloan. Physicians and Patients' Spirituality. AMA Journal of Ethics. 2009, 11(10): 804-815.

22   George D. Pozgar. Legal and ethical issues for health professionals. 2020 by Jones & Bartlett Learning. PP 1-53.

23   Andrew Papanikitas. Crash course, Medical Ethics and Sociology. Second edition. 2013 Elsevier Ltd. PP 1-11.

24   Henk ten Have, Gordijn B. The diversity of bioethics. Med Health Care Philos. 2013 Nov;16(4):635-7.

25 Matti Háyry. A Defense of Ethical Relativism. February 2005Cambridge Quarterly of Healthcare Ethics 14(1):7-12.

26 What is Ethical Relativism? - Saint Peter's University. www.saintpeters.edu › faculty-development › files › 2013/03 › Ethical Relativism Full Analysis. Accessed April 14, 2020.

27 Raanan Gillon, Medical ethics: four principles plus attention to scope. BMJ. 1994 Jul 16;309(6948):184-8.

28 Beauchamp TL, Childress JF. Principle of Biomedical ethics 7th ed. Oxford University Press, 2013.

29 World Medical Association. http//www.wma.net. Principle feature of medical ethics [Archived 4 March 2016, retrieved 3 Nov. 2015.

30 Beauchamp TL: The 'four principles' approach to health care ethics. In Principles of Health Care Ethics. Second ed. Wiley; 2007:3–10.

31 Thomas Grote. Philipp Berens. On the ethics of algorithmic decision-making in healthcare. J Med Ethics 2020;46:205–211.

32 Roger Neighbour. Micro-ethics of the general practice consultation. Chapter in Handbook of primary care ethics. 2018 by Taylor & Francis Group. pp 71-79.

33 P Schröder-Bäck, P Duncan, W Sherlaw, et al. Teaching seven principles for public health ethics: towards a curriculum for a short course on ethics in public health programs. BMC Medical Ethics 2014, 15:73.

34 Swedlow A, Johnson G, smithline N., et al. Increased costs and rates of use in the California workers' compensation system as a result of self-referral by physician. N Eng j med 327(21) 1502-6. 1992.

35 Jordan MC. Ethics Manual fourth edition. American college of Physician. Annals internal medicine 128(7): 576-94, 1998.

36   Legislatures, National conference state, legislative news Studies and analysis- national Conference of State Legislatures, www.ncsi.org. Archived from the Original 2010- 02-24.

37   Guldal D. Semin S. The influences of drug companies' advertising programs on physicians. Int J Health Serv. 2000;30(3):585-95.

38   Baumann A, Audibert G, Guibet Lafaye C, et al. Elective non-therapeutic intensive care and the four principles of medical ethics. J Med Ethics. 2013 Mar;39(3):139-42.

39   Rafik Taibjee. Analyzing an ordinary consultation. Chapter in Handbook of primary care ethics. 2018 by Taylor & Francis Group. pp 81-90.

40   Beth A Lown. A social neuroscience–informed model for teaching and practicing compassion in health care. Medical Education. Volume50, Issue3. March 2016. Pages 332-342.

41   Jodi Halpern. Empathy and Patient–Physician Conflicts. Journal of General Internal Medicine. 22 (2007): 696–700.

42   Robert E. Rakel, "Compassion and the Art of Family Medicine: From Osler to Oprah." Journal of the American Board of Family Medicine, 2000, Vol. 13, Issue 6.

43   Patients' rights. WHO. https://www.who.int/genomics/public/patientrights/en/. Accessed on April 10, 2020.

44   The Johns Hopkins Hospital Patient Rights and Responsibilities. https://www.hopkinsmedicine.org/patient_care/patient-rights-responsibilities.html. Accessed April 10, 2020.

45   George D. Pozgar. Legal and ethical issues for health professionals. 2020 by Jones & Bartlett Learning. pp 363-390.

46　Rights and Responsibilities of Patients - Mayo Clinic. www.mayoclinic. org › documents › mcj6256-pdf › doc-20079310. Accessed April 10, 2020.

47　Natalie L. Birkelien. A Strategic Framework for Improving the Patient Experience in Hospitals. Journal of Healthcare Management. 62, 2017: 250–259.

48　Karen Asp. Is your dr. missing the mark? Shape Magazine. March 2013.

49　Catherine A. Marco, Jay M. Brenner, Chadd K. Kraus, et al. Refusal of emergency medical treatment: case studies and ethical foundations. Ann Emerg Med. 2017;70:696-703.

50　Martín Hevia, Daniela Schnidrig. Terminal Patients and the Right to Refuse Medical Treatment in Argentina. Health and Human Rights. Vol. 18, No. 2, Special Section: Universal Health Coverage and Human Rights (December 2016), pp. 247-250.

51　Thomas Lundmark. Surgery by an unauthorized surgeon as a battery. Cleveland State University. Journal of Law and Health. 1996. https:// engagedscholarship.csuohio.edu/jlh. Accessed April 10, 2020.

52　Nicola Brennan, Rebecca Barnes, Mike Calnan, et al. Trust in the health-care provider–patient relationship: a systematic mapping review of the evidence base. International Journal for Quality in Health Care vol. 25 no. 6. PP 682–688.

53　Jean Drage. New Zealand's National Health and Disability Advocacy Service: A successful model of advocacy. Health and Human Rights Vol. 14, No. 1 (June 2012), pp. 53-63.

54　Kathleen Isaac, Jennifer Hay, Erica Lubetkin. Incorporating Spirituality in Primary Care. J Relig Health. 2016 Jun; 55(3): 1065–1077.

55   Aaron Saguil, Karen Phelps. The Spiritual Assessment. Am Fam Physician. 2012 Sep 15;86(6):546-550.

56   Mark P. Aulisio, Robert M. Arnold, Stuart J. Youngner. Health Care Ethics Consultation: Nature, Goals, and Competencies. Ann Intern Med. 2000;133:59-69.

57   NHS Patient Choice leaflet. www.nhs.uk › NHSEngland › patient-choice › Documents › patient-choice-leaflet.pdf. Accessed April 10, 2020.

58   Michel Daher. Patient Rights. Encyclopedia of Global Bioethics. DOI 10.1007/978-3-319-05544-2_329-1.

59   Trisha Torrey. Your responsibilities as a patient. https://www.verywellhealth.com/patients-responsibilities-2615386. Accessed April 21, 2020.

60   HM Evans. Do patients have duties? J Med Ethics 2007;33:689–694.

61   Patient Responsibilities. AMA Principles of Medical Ethics: I, IV, VI. https://www.ama-assn.org/delivering-care/ethics/patient-responsibilities. Accessed April 21, 2020.

62   Daphne Miller. Why do my patients keep secrets from me? I only want to help them. March 14, 2011. https://www.washingtonpost.com/national/why-do-my-patients-keep-secrets-from-me-i-only-want-to-help-them/2011/03/02/ABYo9uV_story.html. Accessed April 21, 2020.

63   Lauren Vogel. Why do patients often lie to their doctors? CMAJ. Volume 191. Issue 4. P E115.

64   Jenny L. Donovan. Patient decision making: The missing ingredient in compliance research. International Journal of Technology, 1995: 11(3) pp. 443-455.

65 Jane Runzheimer, Linda Johnson Larsen. Medical Ethics for Dummies. John Wiley & Sons 2010.

66 Conrad Fischer, Caterina Oneto. USMLE Medical Ethics. 2006 by Kaplan Publishing, a division of Kaplan, Inc. pp 11-18.

67 George D. Pozgar. Legal and ethical issues for health professionals. 2020 by Jones & Bartlett Learning. pp 282-304.

68 Sandra G. Boodman. Patients Lose When Doctors Can't Do Good Physical Exams. Kaiser Health News • Health & Science • May 20, 2014. https://khn.org/news/patients-lose-when-doctors-do-not-perform-physical-exams-correctly/. Accessed April 23, 2020.

69 Marianne Maumus. The ethics of opiate use and misuse from a hospitalist's perspective. The Ochsner Journal, 2015, 15:124–126.

70 Kirschner N, Ginsburg J, Sulmasy LS. Health and Public Policy Committee of the American College of Physicians. Prescription drug abuse: executive summary of a policy position paper from the American College of Physicians. Ann Intern Med. 2014 Feb 4;160(3):198.

71 Robert D. Truog. Patients and doctors — the evolution of a relationship. n engl j med. February 16, 2012. 366;7.

72 Maatouk-Bürmann B, Ringel N, Spang J, et al. Improving patient centered communication: results of a randomized controlled trial. Patient Educ Couns. 2016;99(1):117-124.

73 Boissy A, Windover AK, Bokar, et al. Communication skills training for physicians improves patient satisfaction. J Gen Intern Med. 2016;31(7):755-761.

74   Lisa S. Rotenstein, Robert S. Huckman, Neil W. Wagle. Making patients and doctors happier — the potential of patient-reported outcomes. N Engl J Med 2017; 377;14.

75   Basch E. Patient-reported outcomes —harnessing patients' voices to improve clinical care. N Engl J Med 2017; 376: 105-8.

76   Albert W. Wu, Roxanne E. Jensen, Claudia Salzberg, Claire Snyder. Advances in the use of patient reported outcome measures in electronic health records including case studies. Baltimore: Patient Centered Outcomes Research Institute, November 7, 2013.

77   Baumhauer JF. Patient-reported outcomes — are they living up to their potential? N Engl J Med 2017; 377: 6-9.

78   Shanafelt TD, Boone S, Tan L, et al. Burnout and satisfaction with work-life balance among US physicians relative to the general US population. Arch Intern Med 2012; 172: 1377-85.

79   Dyrbye LN, Shanafelt TD. Physician burnout: a potential threat to successful health care reform. JAMA 2011; 305: 2009-10.

80   Gelareh Biazar, Kourosh Delpasand, Farnoush Farzi, et al. Breaking bad news: a valid concern among clinicians. Iran J Psychiatry 2019; 14: 3: 198-202.

81   Sarah M. Hilkert, Colleen M. Cebulla, Shelly Gupta Jain, et al. Breaking bad news: a communication competency for ophthalmology training programs. Surv Ophthalmol. 2016 ; 61(6): 791–798.

82   Kimberley R. Monden, Lonnie Gentry, Thomas R. Cox. Delivering bad news to patients. Baylor University Medical Center Proceedings. 2016;29(1):101–102.

83 Buckman R. Communication skills in palliative care: a practical guide. Neurol Clin 2001;19(4):989–1004.

84 Fine RL. Personal choices—communication among physicians and patients when confronting critical illness. Tex Med 1991;87(9):76–82.

85 Edmund G. Howe. When, if ever, should military physicians violate a military order to give medical obligations higher priority? Military medicine, 2015,180, 11:1118.

86 Michael L Gross. Military Medical Ethics. 2003 Cambridge Quarterly of Healthcare Ethics 22(1):92-109.

87 Monica Van Such, Robert Lohr, Thomas Beckman, James M. Naessens. Extent of diagnostic agreement among medical referrals. J Evaluation in Clinical Practice. 2017, 23(4). 870-874.

88 Dieter Grob, Anne F. Mannion. The patient's perspective on complications after spine surgery. Eur Spine J. August 2009, Volume 18, Issue 3, pp 380 – 385.

89 Fritzell P, Hägg O, Nordwall A. Complications in lumbar fusion surgery for chronic low back pain: comparison of three surgical techniques used in a prospective randomized study. A report from the Swedish Lumbar Spine Study Group. Eur Spine J. 2003 Apr;12(2):178-89.

90 Simisade Adedeji, Daniel K. Sokol, Thomas Palser, et al. Ethics of Surgical Complications. World J Surg. 2009 Apr;33(4):732-7.

91 M. S. Pandit, Shobha Pandit. Medical negligence: Coverage of the profession, duties, ethics, case law, and enlightened defense - A legal perspective. Indian J Urol. 2009 Jul-Sep; 25(3): 372–378.

92 Muditha Vidanapathirana. What Do We Know About Medical Negligence? Glob J Nurs Forensic Stud 2016, 1:3.

93   Ten facts on patient safety. https://www.who.int/features/factfiles/patient_safety/en/. Accesses April 15, 2020.

94   Kangasniemi M, Vaismoradi M, Jasper M, et al. Ethical issues in patient safety: Implications for nursing management. Nurs Ethics. 2013 Dec;20(8):904-16.

95   Zahedi F, Sanjari M, Aala M, et al. The code of ethics for nurses. Iran J Public Health. 2013 Jan 1;42(Supple1):1-8.

96   Cecil A. King. Clinical Ethics: Patient and Provider Safety. AORN journal. Dec. 2017. 106(6): pp548-551.

97   Motilal Chandu Tayade, Shashank D. Dalvi. Fundamental ethical issues in unnecessary surgical procedures. J Clin Diagn Res. 2016 Apr; 10(4): JE01–JE04.

98   Philip F. Stahel, Todd F. Vander Heiden, Fernando J. Kim. Why do surgeons continue to perform unnecessary surgery? Patient Safety in Surgery (2017) 11:1.

99   Alexis Black. Unnecessary surgery exposed! Why 60% of all surgeries are medically unjustified and how surgeons exploit patients to generate profits. https://www.naturalnews.com/012291_unnecessary_surgery_hysterectomies.html#ixzz413ZjjTti. Accessed April 12, 2020.

100 Silverberg LI. Survey of medical ethics in US medical schools: a descriptive study. J Am Osteopath Assoc. 2000 Jun;100(6):373-8.

101 JM Mercola. Doctors perform thousands of unnecessary surgeries: are you getting one of them? http://articles.mercola.com/sites/articles/archive/2013/07/10/unnecessary-surgeries.aspx. Accessed April 23, 2020.

102 Goldie J, Schwartz L, Mc Connachie A, et al. Impact of a new course on students' potential behavior on encountering ethical dilemmas. Med Educ. 2001;35:295–302.

103 Leape LL. Unnecessary surgery. Health Serv Res. 1989;24(3):351–407.

104 Nancy E. Epstein, Donald C. Hood. "Unnecessary" spinal surgery: A prospective 1-year study of one surgeon's experience. Surg Neurol Int. 2011; 2: 83.

105 Medtronic spending less on building, and more on selling? www.forbes.com › sites › greatspeculations › 2019/12/03. Accessed on April 18, 2020.

106 Eric Swanson. The commercialization of plastic surgery. Aesthetic Surgery Journal, 2013:33(7) 1065–1068.

107 Hammond DC. The BREAST-Q: further validation in independent clinical samples (discussion). Plast Reconstr Surg. 2012;129:303-304.

108 Kansas State Board of Healing Arts. Statute 65-2837. http://www.ksbha.org/statutes/healingartsact.shtml. Accessed April 18, 2020.

109 Missouri General Assembly. Missouri revised statutes. Statute 334.100. https://law.justia.com/codes/missouri/2011/titlexxii/chapter334/section334100/. Accessed April 18, 2020.

110 American Society of Plastic Surgeons. Article XVI: accredited surgical facilities. https://www1.plasticsurgery.org/search/?ref=/for-medical-professionals/join-asps&q=ASPS-Bylaws. Accessed April 18, 2020.

111 Michael J Kuhar, Dorthie Cross. Collegial ethics: Supporting our colleagues. Science and Engineering Ethics (2013), volume 19, pp 677–684.

112 Michael J. Kuhar. On Blacklisting in Science. Science and Engineering Ethics (2008) volume 14, pp 301–303.

113 Lubalin JS, Matheson JL. The fallout: what happens to whistleblowers and those accused but exonerated of scientific misconduct? Sci Eng Ethics. 1999 Apr;5(2):229-50.

114 T Thirumoorthy. The professional role of the doctor as a colleague – Cultivating healthy collegiality, the forgotten pillar of medical professionalism. SMA News July 2012.

115 Antony Garelick, Leonard Fagin. Doctor to doctor: getting on with colleagues. Advances in Psychiatric Treatment (2004), vol. 10, 225–232.

116 Difficult colleagues. PSS information guide. www.rcpsych.ac.uk › default-source › members › supporting-you › pss. Accessed April 10, 2020.

117 Good Medical Practice: A Code of Conduct for Doctors in Australia. http\\ ama.com.au › files › documents › AMC_Code_of_Conduct_July_2009.pdf. Accessed April 10, 2020.

118 Joseph P. Castlen, David J. Cote, Marike L. D. Broekman. The Ethics of Funding Innovation: Who Should Pay? Chapter in Ethics of Innovation in Neurosurgery. Springer 2019. PP 75-81.

119 Lakdawalla D, Malani A, Reif J. The insurance value of medical innovation. National Bureau of Economic Research Working Paper. 2015.

120 M Bhandari, J W. Busse, D Jackowski, et al. Association between industry funding and statistically significant pro-industry findings in medical and surgical randomized trials. CMAJ 2004;170(4):477-80.

121 Lundh A, Lexchin J, Mintzes B, et al. Industry sponsorship and research outcome. Cochrane Database Syst Rev. 2017;2:MR000033.

122 Pratt B, Hyder AA. Fair resource allocation to health research: priority topics for bioethics scholarship. Bioethics. 2017;31(6):454–66.

123 Orrell K, Yankanah R, Heon E, Wright JG. A small grant funding program to promote innovation at an academic research hospital. Can J Surg. 2015;58(5):294–5.

124 America Research. U.S. Investments in Medical and Health Research and Development, 2013-2016. 2016. p. 3–6.

125 Kaiser J. Biomedical research policy. NIH funding shifts with disease lobbying, study suggests. Science. 2012;338(6104):181.

126 The Lancet Oncology. Mind the gap: charity and crowd funding in health care. Lancet Oncol. 2017;18(3):269.

127 Ethics Committee. Greater Manchester Combined Authority. https://www.greatermanchester-ca.gov.uk/what-we-do/police-plus-fire/ethics-committee/. Accessed April 12, 2020.

128 Ethics Committee of the British Psychological Society. https://www.bps.org.uk/who-we-are/ethics-committee. Accessed April 12, 2020.

129 Linda Ray. What Are the Roles of Ethics Committees? https://bizfluent.com/how-8146549-make-ethical-decisions-management.html. Accessed April 12, 2020.

130 Ethical committees | Karolinska Institute. https://ki.se/en/km/ethical-committees. Accessed April 12, 2020.

131 Ethics committee (European Union). https://en.wikipedia.org/wiki/Ethics_committee_(European_Union). Accessed April 12, 2020.

132 NHS Research Ethics Committee. https://www.hra.nhs.uk/approvals-amendments/what-approvals-do-i-need/research-ethics-committee-review/. Accessed April 12, 2020.

133 Nayan Lamba, Marike L. D. Broekman. Research ethics: when innovation is clearly research. Chapter in Ethics of Innovation in Neurosurgery. Springer 2019. PP 143-150.

134 Emanuel EJ, Wendler D, Grady C. What makes clinical research ethical? JAMA. 2000 May 24-31;283(20):2701-11.

135 Adil E. Shamoo, David B. Resnik. Responsible conduct of research. Third edition. Oxford University Press 2015.

136 Jackson B. The Bristol enquiry report: care in the operating theatre and the "learning curve". www.bristol-inquiry.org.uk/final_report/annex_a/chapter_14_15.htm. Accessed April 20, 2020.

137 AN Hopper, MH Jamison, W G Lewis. Learning curves in surgical practice. Postgrad Med J. 2007 Dec; 83(986): 777–779.

138 Bridgewater B, Grayson AD, Au J, et al. Improving mortality of coronary surgery over first four years of independent practice: retrospective examination of prospectively collected data from 15 surgeons. BMJ (Clin Res ed) 2004;329:421.

139 Ramsay CR, Grant AM, Wallace SA, et al. Assessment of the learning curve in health technologies. A systematic review. Int J Technol Assess Health Care 2000;16:1095–108.

140 Lynda Charters. Caution key when embracing new technologies in clinical practice. Ophthalmology Times. Vol 45 No 5. March 2020.

Ethics In Spine Surgery

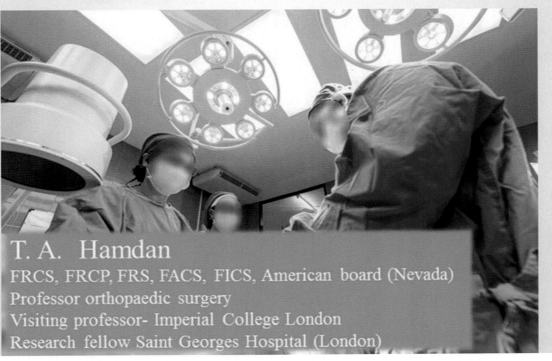

T. A. Hamdan
FRCS, FRCP, FRS, FACS, FICS, American board (Nevada)
Professor orthopaedic surgery
Visiting professor- Imperial College London
Research fellow Saint Georges Hospital (London)

Definition of ethics

- Moral principles that govern a person's behavior or the conducting of activity
- The branch of knowledge that deals with moral principle
- Ethics or moral philosophy is a branch of philosophy that involves systemizing defending and recommending concept of right and wrong conduct
- Cambridge Dictionary definition of a system of accepted beliefs that control behavior especially such a system based on moral

Probably the best definition is of medical dictionary:

➡A branch of philosophy dealing with values pertaining to human contact

➡Considering the rightness and wrongness of action and the goodness or badness of the motives and ends of such actions i.e. systematic rules of principles governing right contact.

The four corners of ethics

1. Respect for autonomy
2. Beneficence
3. Non maleficence
4. Justice

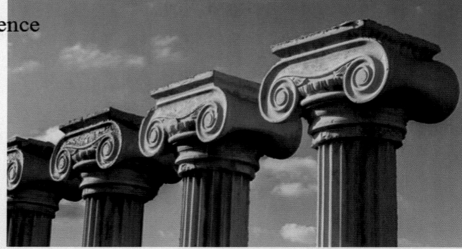

And I confidently respect for patient's dignity

Codes for ethics

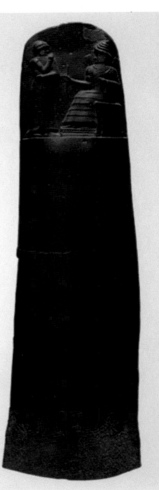

- Hippocratic Oath
- Hammurabi code 1750 B.C.
- Declaration of genera
- Nuremberg code
- World Medical Association
- Declaration of Helsinki
- Code of ethics: A. M. Association and American orthopaedic association and others

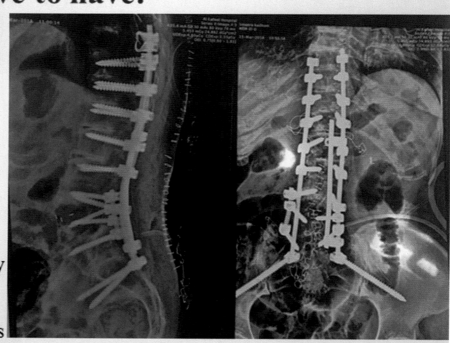

To be competent spinal surgeon, you have to have:

- Skills
- Judgment
- Ethics
- Training
- Experience
- Loss of Ego
- Do it well.
- Do it differently
- Or don't at all
- (John D. Davis 2003)

Judgment

- The ability to assimilate symptoms, signs, imaging, investigations and make sound decisions
- Hard to teach
- More than knowledge
- Not always easy to achieve
- The responsibility to act in the best interest of the patients

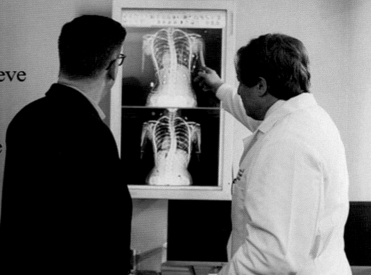

Clinical judgment

➡ Comes as a priority

➡ Beware of false positive investigation and imaging

➡ The decision to operate depends on clinical judgment to be confirmed by investigations and imaging

➡ Always decision before incision

The humanitarian handling

- First visit either salt in the wound or lifelong friendship
- Humanitarianism:
- Is the active belief in the value you of human life?
- All humans deserve respect and dignity and should be treated as such
- The principle of humanitarian action are humanity, neutrality, independence, and impartiality, all people have equal dignity
- Big smile, smooth welcoming words followed by careful listening and gentle physical examination

Informed consent (written)

- Permission granted in full knowledge of the possible consequence
- Typically what is given by a patient to doctor for treatment with knowledge of possible risks and benefits
- The medical provider must be disclose information on the treatment, test, or procedure in question
- This collaborative decision making process is an ethical and legal obligation of the health care provider
- Can others sign the consent?
- Implied consent

Communication skills

- How to deliver the bad news
- Simply the ability to transfer messages in a smooth and gentle way
- ? What about sad news
- How to improve clinical skills
- Respect and appreciation
- Listen activity
- Ask questions and paraphrase
- Eyes contact
- Pay attention to   body language
- Pay away devices, like cell phone
- Watch your tone
- Smile and have positive attitude

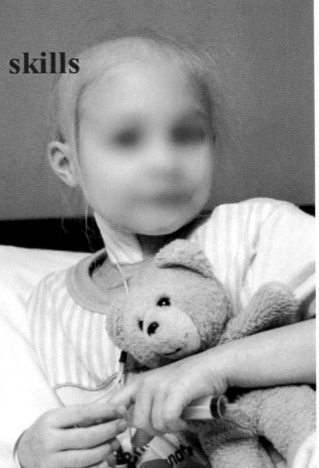

Investigation and imaging (not exchange of benefit)

- ➡ Mutual benefit in referral
- ➡ Deceptive guidance
- ➡ Very much hateful
- ➡ Probably harmful to the patient in some occasion

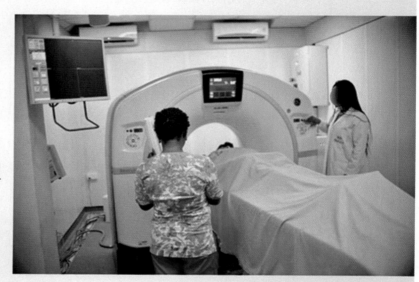

Timing of surgery depends on the pattern of disease

➡ Emergency
➡ Elective
➡ Semi- emergency
➡ Time Factor is very vital
➡ Unnecessary delay is unethical and no reason to accept

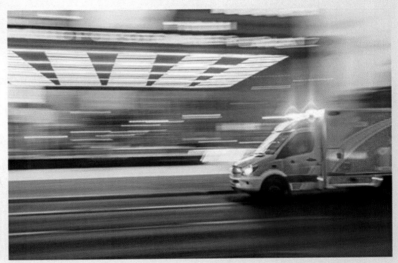

- What is never accepted, is no surgery or delayed surgery because of financial issue
- Timely treatment is mandatory for certain spinal pathology
- Balance between unnecessary haste and unreasonable delay
- No substitute for the experience
- Attention to the result or clinical examination
- Imaging and investigation
- No hurry, take your time
- Consult if required

Treatment offered

- There must be a limit for conservative treatment
- We have to know when to stop conservative treatment
- Do not give narcotics and non- narcotics without identifying the underlying cause or causes
- Least possible of narcotics, steroids, and hormones
- When to   operate on emergency conditions
- The pattern of treatment should be far away from cost wise and the pressure or companies

Prescribing narcotics and other medications

- Not to induce dependency or addiction
- In my mind the side effect
- Cost wise
- Absolute indication
- No analgesia before identifying the cause

Appointing proxy

- Ask the patient to do it
- Because of unforeseen situation at the time I'm of operation
- Urgent decision is required intraoperative

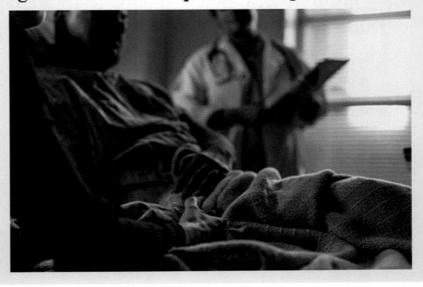

Conflict of interest

- Tell the truth as it is
- Be frank and honest as expected from you
- Mention if you have received financial support from drug companies, medical equipment and spinal implant companies

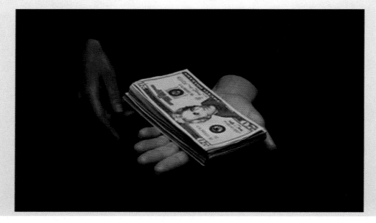

Ethics after complications and bad outcome

- Painful situation. We have to face
- Hopefully the surgeon is not part of the complications, if so better admit
- Try to hug your patient, don't try to push him away
- After the utmost service possible
- Be very helpful from all points of View
- Certainly it is very unethical to leave him alone in the wind

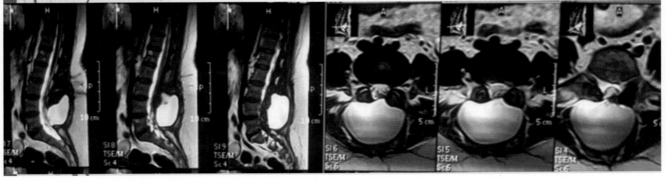

The effects of funding innovation

➡ Who should pay?
➡ Examine the source of funding
➡ Patient self-payment
➡ Insurance involvement
➡ Industry funding
➡ Philanthropy: individual donation, patient support groups, charitable Foundation, or other sources
➡ Academic/ institutional support
➡ Government grants
➡ Crow funding website: life patient funding, should be avoided
➡ No matter where the money comes from innovation will inherently come with some degree of pressure for certain results (Castlen etal. 2019)

Cost aware

- It's patient money- not our money
- Resources are Limited
- All diagnostic tests and treatment are costy and have risks
- Spine surgeon is very expensive surgery
- Follow up is not without cost

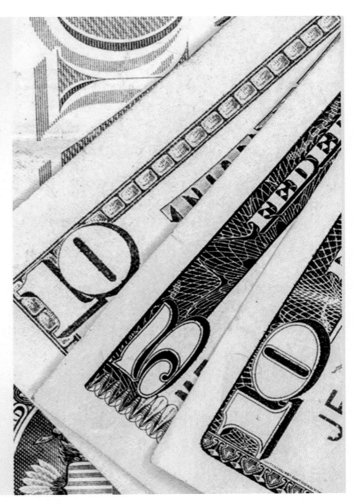

Second opinion

- Two brains are much better than one
- You will never lose by getting second opinion
- Consult colleagues, you will share with their brains
- Free of cost
- Patient will respect you
- Much better than doing harm to the patient is to get second opinion
- Second opinion will dissolve your anxiety and apprehension and strengthen the relation with colleagues

Handling the seriously ill and terminally ill patient

- One of the most things to go through as a spine surgeon
- Need care in 3 areas
- Physical comfort: i.e. proper positioning
- Emotional support: i.e. help to manage mental and emotional stress
- Spiritual needs: i.e. Perform certain prayers
- Supporting the family member to help the patient and to be helped
- What is required from the surgeon end?

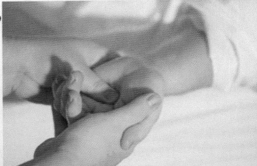

Colleague's relations

- Be Friendly, supportive and helpful
- You meet him every day, probably more than your family and certainly more than your patients
- Part of your job is to rectify his mistakes
- Tell him reconstructive remarks, and exchange experience with him
- Tell him about his negative points, but never tell the patient about his mistakes
- The difficult situation? (I hate to face it)

Unnecessary surgery

- Worldwide, every year millions of people go under the knife because of unnecessary surgery
- May endure suffering
- Shelling thousands of Dollars
- The estimated figure all over the world varies from 30-70% (Lepe LL 1992)
- Simply done because for profit or corporate targets of the hospital
- The rate of medical harm occurring in US is estimated to be over 40000 harmful and/or lethal error every year (Dr. Mercoln 2016)

Training the junior staff

- They have the wright to improve their Technical skills
- Should be under strict supervision
- Better not to leave the follow-up for them

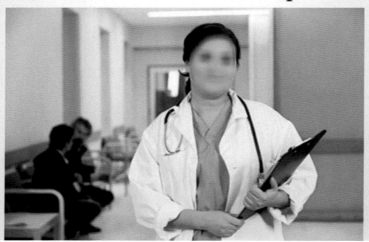

Commercialization of carrier

- The organization of something in away intended to make a profit

- The process for developing or organizing something in order to make as much money as possible

- Real marketing. Sometimes far away from reality and the humanity

- This is particularly finished pine Surgery. New implants, fixators, medications

- Convincing spine surgeon for exchange of benefits (mutual benefit)

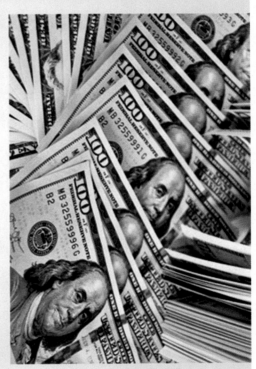

The relation between the spine surgeon, pharmaceutical and medical device industries

➡ Even indirect relationships with industry can compromised patient care

➡ The presence of company representatives in theatre can cause favorability towards particular company

➡ Choose the best fixator, Implants, or medicine for your patients and avoid bias towards the representative

➡ Don't let them buy your brain or your ethics

➡ Never let the business interest impact on your decision making

Research ethics

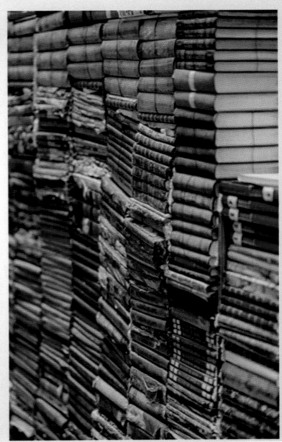

➡ History confirmed the aerocities and violation of human dignity because of unethical research

➡ Structured ethical frameworks serves the research very much and there is a desperate need for this

➡ Honesty in research

Research ethics

Emanuel et al. (2000) described 7 requirements for ethical research:

1. Social and scientific value
2. Scientific validity
3. Fair subject selection
4. Favorable risk-benefit ratio
5. Independent review
6. Informed consent
7. Respect for both initial and enrolled subjects

The ethics committee

➡ Mandatory in every Institutes, Hospitals, universities, even in funding companies and others

➡ It is governing center has the voice to say yes or no depending on solid bases

➡ Should consist of pioneers and experienced personnel, ethics supporters

➡ Rejections or acceptance, depends on how useful and how harmful the depending on solid ethical background

Finally

- Ethics is particularly required spinal   practice
- Always keep yourself away from the pressure of companies
- Colleagues relationships is vital
- Patients benefit comes on the top or everything
- Big gain nothing to lose for getting second opinion
- No research without ethical background
- Informed consent and conflict of interest are mandatory
- Treatment design should solely serve the patient interest

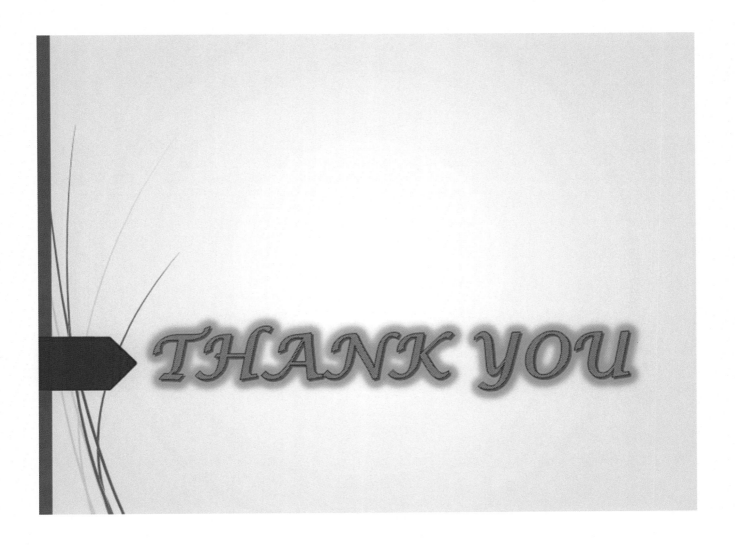

Printed in the United States
By Bookmasters